Peter Kühn, MD   ·   Clemens Lang   ·   Franz Wiesbauer, MD MPH

ECG MASTERY

The Simplest Way to
Learn the ECG

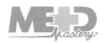

ECG Mastery: The Simplest Way to Learn the ECG

by Peter Kühn, MD, Clemens Lang, and Franz Wiesbauer, MD MPH

ISBN: 978-3-9503944-0-5

Cover and interior design: Philipp Gärtner
Layout: Brigitte Mair
Editor and proofreader: Mary L. Tod, PhD, ELS
Project manager: Bonnie Bills

http://www.medmastery.com

Table of Contents

Introduction   1

An innovative approach to mastering the ECG   2

How to get the most out of this book   2

Other learning resources—including a free e-book!   3

About the authors   4

Acknowledgements   5

Level 1:   **Deconstructing the ECG curve—the components of the tracing**   7

Key concepts   8

Identifying the components of the QRS complex   9

Example: identifying P waves, QRS complexes, and T waves   9

Quiz section   10

Level 2:   **Interval (time) and amplitude (voltage) measurements**   13

The ECG grid   14

The Y-axis—amplitude measurement   14

The X-axis—time measurement   15

Measuring intervals   15

Quiz section   17

Level 3:   **When the timing is off—the foundations of interval interpretation**   21

Duration of the P wave   22

Duration of the PR interval   23

QRS duration   24

Quiz section   25

Level 4:   **The precordial leads—what nobody ever tells you**   29

How to place the precordial leads   30

How to find and count the intercostal spaces correctly   31

What anatomical regions are depicted by what leads?   31

The normal pattern   33

The R/S ratio ("R to S ratio")   33

Quiz section   37

Level 5:   **The chest leads—100% confidence**   39

A normal ECG   40

Patterns in abnormal ECGs   40

Quiz section   44

Level 6: What you really need to know about ventricular hypertrophy   **49**

Key concepts   50

The Sokolow index   51

Now, let's turn to right ventricular hypertrophy...   52

Quiz section   53

Level 7: ST depression and T negativity—a simple approach   **59**

Key concepts   60

The different forms of ST depressions   61

Patterns of negative T waves (also known as T-wave inversions)   62

Quiz section   63

Level 8: What everybody ought to know about myocardial infarction and the QRS complex   **69**

Drowning in negativity   70

Pathologic or not pathologic—that is the question   72

Two important tricks for your toolbox   74

Quiz section   76

Level 9: Inferior wall myocardial infarction—pearls and pitfalls   **81**

The limb leads   82

Looking at mirror images   84

Q-wave and non−Q-wave infarctions   85

Please welcome ... the ECG cookbook!   85

Quiz section   87

Level 10: Acute coronary syndromes—mastering the ST segment   **91**

The acute coronary syndromes   92

Pathways I and II—ACS with ST elevation   94

Pathway III—ACS without ST elevation   94

Pathway IV—Prinzmetal angina: a special case   95

Perimyocarditis   95

Vagotonia   96

Quiz section   99

Level 11: The ECG trio—cardiac axis, atrial hypertrophy, and low-voltage   **105**

    The shocking truth about the cardiac axis   106

    Atrial hypertrophy   116

    Low voltage   117

    Quiz section   120

Level 12: A short story about electrolytes and heart rate   **127**

    Hyperkalemia and hypokalemia   128

    Hypocalcemia and hypercalcemia   129

    Heart rate quick tip   130

    Quiz section   133

Level 13: Rhythm 101—the sinus rhythm   **139**

    Criteria for sinus rhythm   140

    Quiz section   143

Quiz solutions: **151**

    Level 1   152

    Level 2   154

    Level 3   157

    Level 4   160

    Level 5   161

    Level 6   166

    Level 7   172

    Level 8   177

    Level 9   181

    Level 10   186

    Level 11   192

    Level 12   298

    Level 13   206

Index   **216**

Introduction

Introduction

In this section you'll learn how to get the most out of this book, as well as how to download all the resources that come with it—including a free copy of the next book in this series!

An innovative approach to mastering the ECG

Welcome to *ECG Mastery: The Simplest Way to Learn the ECG*, a hands-on workbook designed to make learning the ECG easy, effective, and fun. We created this book to address the concerns we kept hearing from ECG students (and doctors seeking to upgrade their ECG skills!)—that ECG books and training courses focus more on theory than on practice, that people want to learn from real-world cases, that learning the ECG is unnecessarily complicated and, well, not very much fun. We think learning the ECG doesn't have to be that way, so we created this book. Here's why we think you'll like it:

- It leaves out the jargon and sticks to the hands-on information that's really important.
- Dozens of quizzes based on actual cases allow you to practice what you've learned.
- Visuals on every page help you grasp the key concepts.
- You'll come to truly understand the ECG without memorizing anything.

How to get the most out of this book

In this book, you'll learn the basics of the ECG language. After going through it, you'll be able to recognize many common and dangerous diseases. You'll learn quickly and effortlessly, and when you're done, you'll be able to follow a case discussion among your colleagues and begin using the ECG in your daily clinical practice. Each section starts out with a brief explanation of the basics, followed by a selection of hand-picked ECG cases and quizzes. (Solutions to the quizzes are at the end of the book.) These cases are intended to reinforce what you have learned in each section.

You'll get most out of this book if you go through the chapters in a sequential order. Each chapter prepares you for the next one.

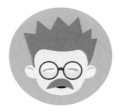 *Reading the ECG is like riding a bike—once you've learned how to do it, you won't forget it.*

Other learning resources—including a free e-book!

This book is part of the ECG Mastery program from Medmastery, which includes books, e-books, and interactive online courses.

Our ECG program is subdivided into a Yellow Belt for beginners, a Blue Belt for the moderately advanced, and a Black Belt for very advanced folks. This book is a companion to our Yellow Belt online training course. (Don't worry, though; this book was designed as a standalone training resource—in fact, thousands of people have learned from our books alone.) It covers all the basic concepts you need to know to start using the ECG in your daily clinical practice.

Get free access to the Blue Belt book, too!
Medmastery also offers more advanced ECG training, in the form of our Blue Belt course and companion workbook. By purchasing this book, you get free access to the Blue Belt workbook, which focuses entirely on how to assess heart rhythms on the ECG. After going through our Blue Belt training, you'll be able to diagnose 95% of cases without the help of a more senior colleague. To get access to the workbook, just point your web browser to **www.medmastery.com/ECGbook** and type in the code ECG123 !

Additional learning resources

We created additional downloadable learning resources that can be used as pocket references during your day in the clinic. Here they are:

1. The **ECG Cookbook** is a quick reference that will help you to remember the step-by-step diagnostic approach taught in this book.
2. The **Rhythm Cheat Sheet** goes along with our Blue Belt course and workbook. It's a simple stepwise approach for solving almost any rhythm problem.
3. The **Little Black Book of ECG Secrets** is an ECG case collection with links to teaching videos and expert video solutions.

To download these resources, go to **www.medmastery.com/ECGbook** and type in the code **ECG123** !

The ECG Mastery program online

If you are looking for more hands-on practice or more advanced ECG training, ECG Mastery offers interactive, case-based online courses. You can get a feel for the online experience by signing up for a free trial account to the ECG Mastery program at **www.medmastery.com**. On top of our two books, this online course provides you with:

- Hours of video lectures
- Interactive ECG cases
- Video analysis showing how an expert would solve each case
- Access to the Black Belt section, which will bring your ECG skills to an entirely new level.

For a small monthly subscription, you'll get access to the entire ECG Mastery program. We would love to see you inside!

About the authors

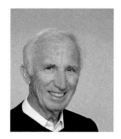

Peter Kühn, MD, is an internist with a specialization in cardiology. He trained at the Medical University of Vienna and the Institute for Muscle Disease in New York City. Professor Kühn has written several ECG books and has decades of teaching experience. He was the head of the cardiology department of the hospital Barmherzige Schwestern in Linz, Austria, between 1976 and 2002.

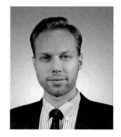

Clemens Lang is a medical student living in Vienna, Austria. Clemens has a passion for new technologies and new ways of teaching. Clemens loves his band, traveling to see as many countries as possible, playing piano, good food, and basketball.

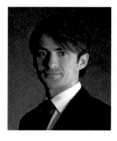

Franz Wiesbauer, MD MPH, is an internist with a specialization in cardiology. He trained at the Medical University of Vienna and The Johns Hopkins University in Baltimore where he was a Fulbright scholar. He is an associate Professor for internal medicine at the Medical University of Vienna.

Acknowledgements

We would like to thank our entire team at Medmastery for their great work. First and foremost, we would like to thank Bonnie Bills for coordinating the production process and for all her thoughtful comments. Secondly, we would like to thank Philipp Gärtner and Brigitte Mair, our designers, for doing a tremendous job creating the visuals and layout for the book, and Mary L. Tod for her sharp and sensitive editing. Lastly, we would like to thank you, our readers, for your feedback, comments, and encouragement.

We'd also like to give a special shout-out to the enthusiastic beta testers and readers who gave us feedback on our ECG Mastery program (including this text) as we developed it:

A. B. Atuchukwu, Abdisalam Abdi, Adedeji Adebayo, MD, Ahmad Shoaib, MD, Amina Durodola, Amr Abdelghany, MD, Besim H Guda, MD, Bulungu Tshinanu, MD, César Ferreira, Daniel Alves, MD, MSc, Farzane Barzkar, Gaurav Kapoor, MD, Georgi Minchev, Godsent Isiguzo, Hassan Almaateeq, Ibrahim Aliyu, Ibrahim Ghazi, MD, Ivana Begic, MD, José Carlos Moreno Samos, MD, Juliaty Eds, Ka Wah-Li, Katya Mollova, Katya Mollova, MD, Keramida Kalliopi MD, MSc, PhD, Kero Wasss, Lola Rakhimdjanova, Maria del Mar, Mehmet K. Çelenk, Michele Escande Orthlieb, Michelle Gagnon, BS, RDCS, RVT, Nato Chubinidze, Nchafatso Obonyo, MD, Osman Ahmed, Peter-Louis Ndifor, Petrica Ciobanca, Rana A Kundu, Rosie Beles, Tarek Mazzawi, Theo Rosales, Tsogzol Dorji, Virgilio de Asa Jr., Yura Mareev, and Zulfiqar Ahmed, MD.

This book is dedicated to all the doctors out there who are striving to become better and better every day. It's your relentless quest for knowledge and mastery that ultimately drives progress in medicine.

Level 1

Deconstructing the ECG curve—
the components of the tracing

"You cannot open a book without learning something."
—Confucius

Deconstructing the ECG curve– the components of the tracing

In this first chapter, you will learn about the different waves on the ECG and how to recognize them.

Key concepts

Your first step is to learn how to identify QRS complexes, T waves, and P waves on a tracing.

The **isoelectric line** is the baseline of the ECG. By definition, it's the line on the ECG during which electrical activity is absent—look for the flat line that connects a T wave to the following P wave. Anything above is positive, anything below is negative.

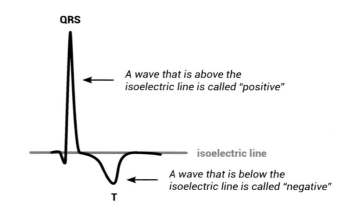

QRS

A wave that is above the isoelectric line is called "positive"

isoelectric line

A wave that is below the isoelectric line is called "negative"

T

Electrical depolarization of the ventricles leads to sharp deflections in the ECG called **QRS complexes**. Every depolarization is followed by a phase of repolarization. Repolarization of the ventricles is represented by the so-called **T waves**. The T wave can be positive or negative.

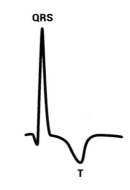

Atrial depolarization is depicted by the **P wave**, which is steeper than the T wave but flatter than the QRS complex. We said that every depolarization is followed by a phase of repolarization. But since atrial repolarization happens at the same time as the QRS complex, it cannot be recognized on the ECG.

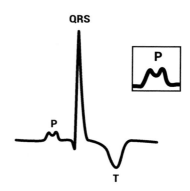

Identifying the components of the QRS complex

There are five concepts that will help you to identify the different components of the QRS complex.

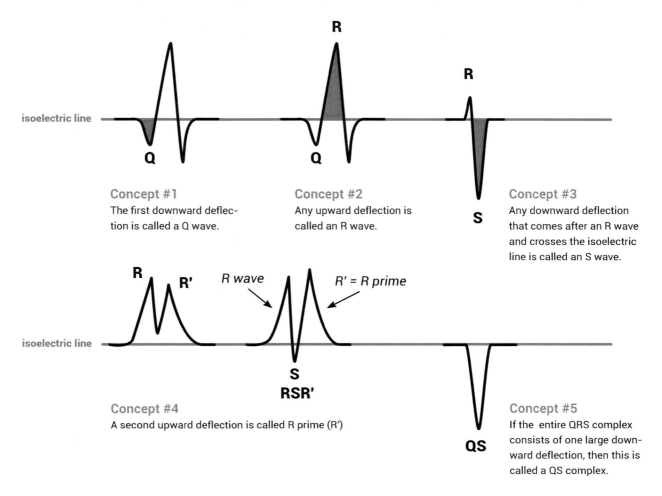

Concept #1
The first downward deflection is called a Q wave.

Concept #2
Any upward deflection is called an R wave.

Concept #3
Any downward deflection that comes after an R wave and crosses the isoelectric line is called an S wave.

Concept #4
A second upward deflection is called R prime (R')

Concept #5
If the entire QRS complex consists of one large downward deflection, then this is called a QS complex.

Example: identifying P waves, QRS complexes, and T waves

Based on the concepts outlined above, we can now identify the P waves, QRS complexes, and T waves in an example exercise. Notice that the second wave is steep and edgy; it has sharper deflections than the other curves and therefore has to be the QRS complex.

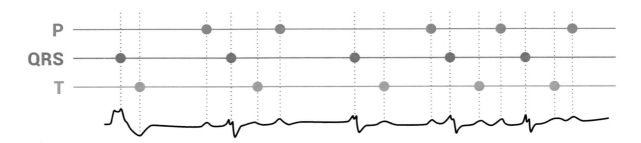

Dotted vertical lines originate from the different waves of the ECG. They intersect with horizontal lines identifying P, QRS, and T. In this example we have already identified the different waves for you.

Level 1

QUIZ SECTION

Now it is your turn. If in doubt, start looking for the QRS complex (focus on sharp deflections!). Also keep in mind that every QRS complex is followed by the T wave after 200 – 400 ms (equivalent to 5 – 10 mm on this ECG paper). In the next step you should already be able to identify the P wave, as the steepness of its deflection is in between that of the QRS and the T waves.

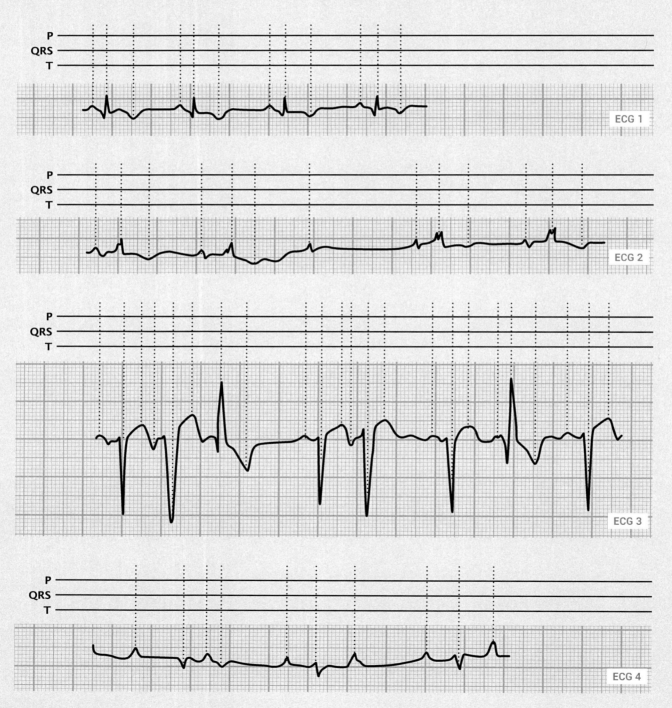

Interval (time) and amplitude (voltage) measurements

"If you can't make a mistake, you can't make anything."
—Marva Collins

Interval (time) and amplitude (voltage) measurements

In this chapter, you will learn about the duration and amplitudes of the various waves and how to measure them.

The ECG grid

You can measure in two dimensions on the ECG paper. The Y-axis shows amplitudes (i.e., voltage), while the X-axis shows time.

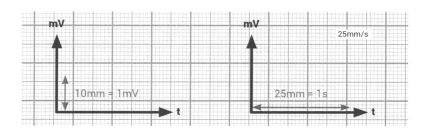

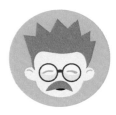

Measuring is not always necessary in order to come up with the right diagnosis. Some diseases just require pattern recognition (e.g., acute myocardial infarction), while others require measurements (e.g., ventricular hypertrophy, bundle branch blocks, etc.).

The Y-axis—amplitude measurement

Amplitude or voltage is measured on the Y-axis; 10 mm represents 1 millivolt (mV) with standard calibration. Occasionally, calibration is set at double standard (20 mm = 1 mV) or half standard (5 mm = 1 mV). However, this is only rarely done. So just remember that 10 mm = 1 mV and you'll be fine in 99.9% of cases.

Here's how you can tell if the ECG is adjusted to standard calibration. Almost every ECG printout also has a rectangular calibration signal on it. If the machine is set to standard calibration (10 mm = 1 mV), this calibration signal will be exactly 10 mm high as shown in the example.

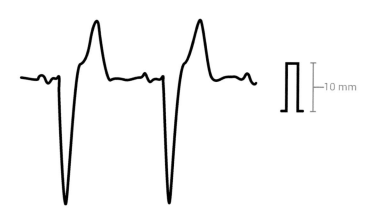

The X-axis—time measurement

Most ECG machines print at a speed of 25 mm per second. Therefore, a 25-mm distance on the X-axis corresponds to a duration of 1 second. So remember:

- 25 mm on the X-axis = 1 second
- 5 mm (large box) on X-axis = 1/5 of a second or 0.2 seconds
- 1 mm (small box) on X-axis = 1/5 of 0.2 seconds or 0.04 seconds

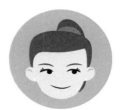

Occasionally, paper speed is set at 50 mm/s in which case all ECG intervals are twice as long as normal (large box = 0.1 s instead of 0.2 s, small box = 0.02 s instead of 0.04 s). So whenever all intervals look too long, check for an increase of paper speed to 50 mm/s.

Measuring intervals

Now it's time to carry out some measurements. The duration of a wave is measured from its initial deviation from the isoelectric line until the point where it returns to the isoelectric line again. The amplitude of the wave is the distance between the isoelectric line and the peak or nadir of that wave.

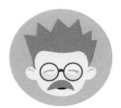

You should try to evaluate and measure each ECG in a systematic way, one step after the other. In later chapters we will introduce such an approach, which we call the "ECG Cookbook."

Here is how to measure the different intervals:

Measurement of P-wave duration starts at the point where the P wave leaves the isoelectric line until it returns to the isoelectric line again.

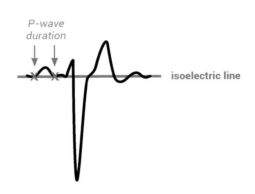

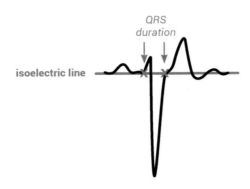

Measurement of QRS duration starts at the point where the QRS complex leaves the isoelectric line until it returns to the isoelectric line again.

Measurement of the QT interval starts at the beginning of the QRS complex until the end of the T wave.

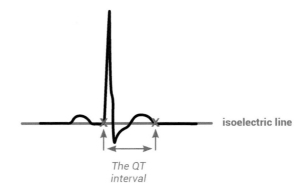

isoelectric line

The QT interval

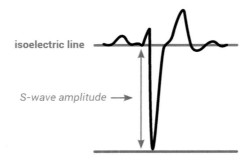

isoelectric line

S-wave amplitude →

Measurement of amplitudes: start measuring at the isoelectric line until the nadir or peak of the wave.

Level 2

QUIZ SECTION

Now it is again your turn; perform the measurements mentioned above.

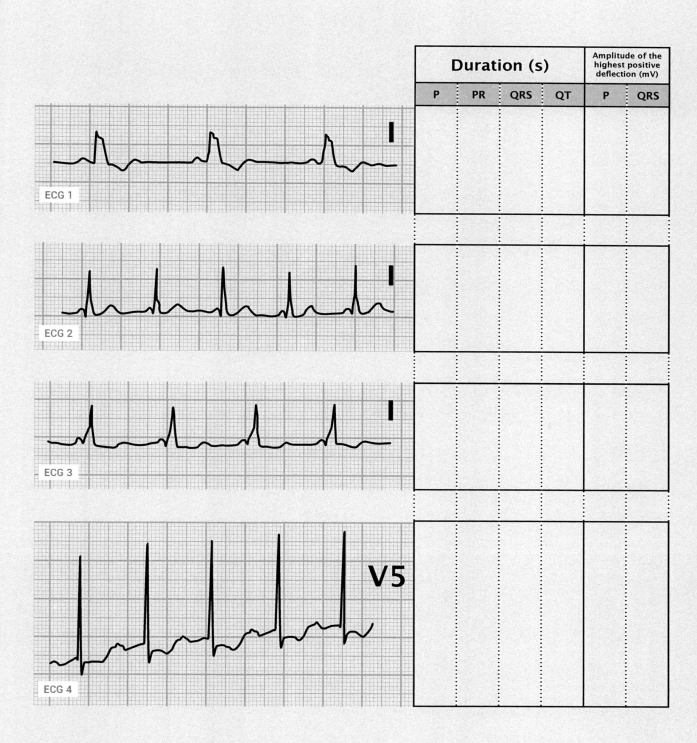

	Duration (s)				Amplitude of the highest positive deflection (mV)	
P	**PR**	**QRS**	**QT**	**P**	**QRS**

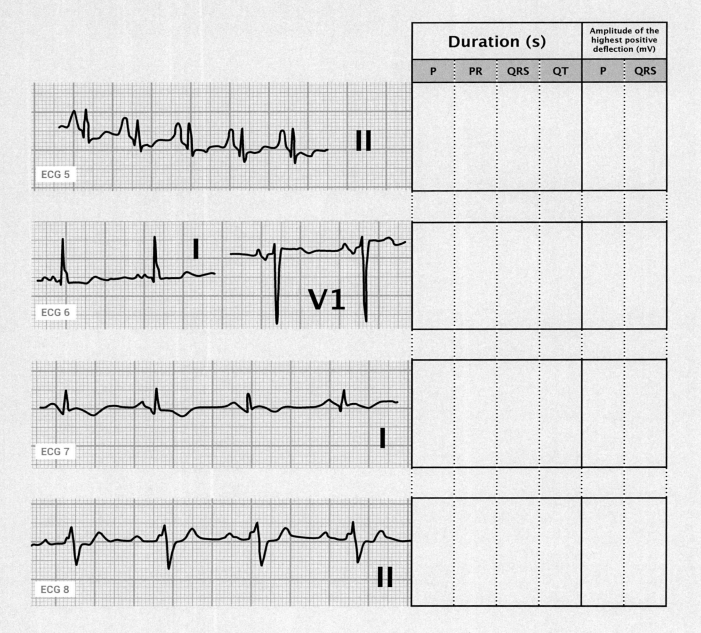

	Duration (s)				Amplitude of the highest positive deflection (mV)	
P	PR	QRS	QT		P	QRS

Level 3

When the timing is off–
the foundations of interval interpretation

*"Tell me and I forget, teach me and I may
remember, involve me and I learn."*
—Benjamin Franklin

When the timing is off—the foundations of interval interpretation

In this chapter, you will learn about the normal values of the different time intervals and what it means if they are longer or shorter than normal.

Duration of the P wave

Depolarization of the atria (i.e., P-wave duration) usually takes **less than 0.10 seconds**. If the left atrium is dilated (enlarged), depolarization takes longer and **P-wave duration will increase to ≥0.12 s**.

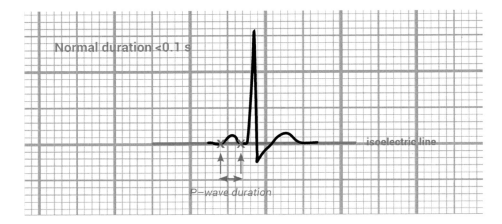

The prolonged P wave seen in atrial enlargement has a "double peak" in lead I and lead II and is called **P mitrale** (see image). You will learn more about this in Level 11.

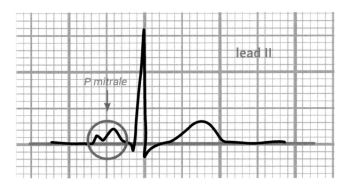

Duration of the PR interval

The **PR interval** represents the duration the impulse takes to travel from the atria to the ventricles. It's measured from the beginning of the P wave until the beginning of the QRS complex. **Normal values** are between **0.12 and 0.2 seconds**. Any duration below or above this range is regarded as abnormal.

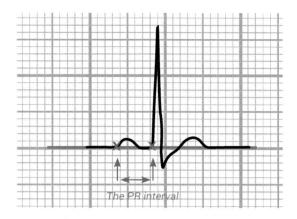

The PR interval

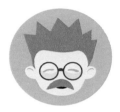

Paradoxically, it's always called a "PR interval," no matter whether the QRS complex starts with a Q or an R wave.

When the PR interval is >0.2 seconds

When the PR interval is longer than 0.2 seconds AND there is a QRS complex after each P wave, we have what is called a **first degree atrioventricular block** (or AV block I), as seen on the image.

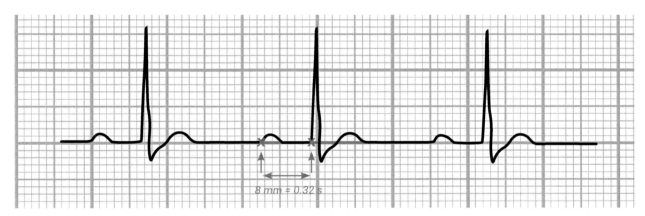

8 mm = 0.32 s

Example of a first degree AV block (AV block I). In this case, the PR interval is 0.32 s and there is a QRS complex after each P wave.

When the PR interval is <0.12 seconds

When the PR interval is shorter than 0.12 seconds, depolarization of the ventricles occurs earlier than normal. This situation is called **preexcitation** (or **preexcitation syndrome**). In these syndromes, an additional bundle conducts the impulse down from the atria to the ventricles. The conduction speed in the additional bundle is faster than in the AV node—so the impulse reaches the ventricles earlier than normal and the PR interval is shortened.

There are two important preexcitation syndromes that you should remember. The **Lown-Ganong-Levine syndrome (LGL syndrome)** is characterized by a QRS complex that immediately follows the P wave. The appearance and duration of the QRS complexes are normal.

The other form of preexcitation is called **Wolff-Parkinson-White syndrome (WPW syndrome)**. A slurred upstroke of the QRS complex immediately follows the P wave; it is also known as a "delta wave," as it resembles the Greek letter delta. The duration of the QRS is usually lengthened to >0.12 s.

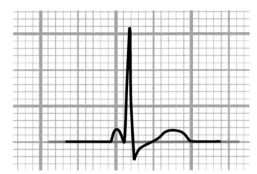

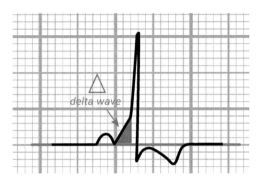

Lown-Ganong-Levine syndrome
= LGL syndrome

- QRS immediately follows the P wave
- QRS looks normal
- QRS duration is normal

Wolff-Parkinson-White syndrome
= WPW syndrome

- QRS immediately follows the P wave
- QRS looks abnormal (delta wave)
- QRS duration >0.12 s

QRS duration

Under normal circumstances, depolarization of the ventricles takes up to 0.10 seconds. Dilatation of the ventricles may cause a slight lengthening of the QRS (>0.1 to <0.12 s). A significantly prolonged **QRS duration of ≥0.12s**, however, indicates that either the right or left bundle branch is blocked. This situation is called a **complete bundle branch block**. You will learn more about it in Level 5.

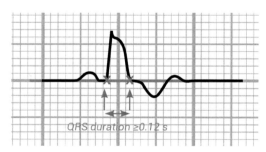

Complete bundle branch block

There are also other reasons for broad QRS complexes. As we have just learned, one such example is the WPW syndrome, in which a delta wave is added at the beginning of the QRS complex. Other reasons will be introduced in later chapters.

Level 3

QUIZ SECTION

The following examples may seem familiar to you, but at this time not only the measurements but also the correct diagnoses are required. Note that there may be more than only one abnormality in a single example!

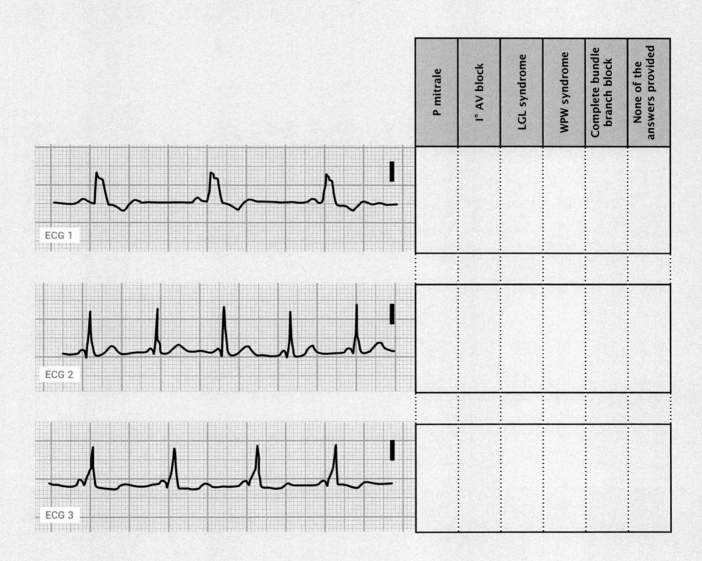

	P mitrale	I° AV block	LGL syndrome	WPW syndrome	Complete bundle branch block	None of the answers provided
ECG 1						
ECG 2						
ECG 3						

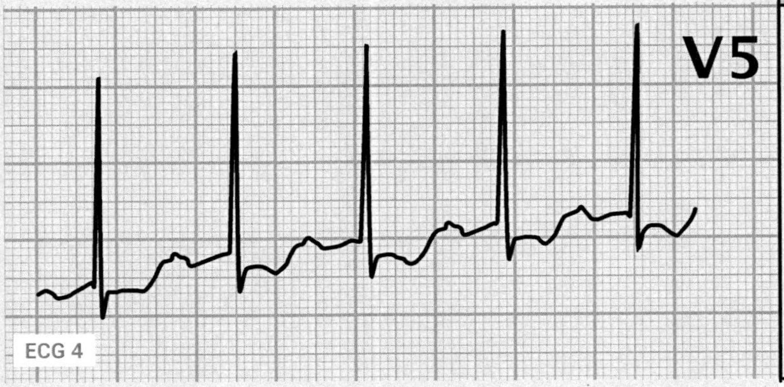

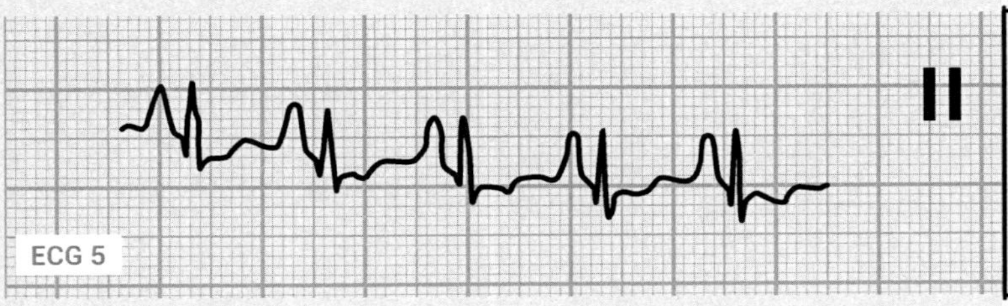

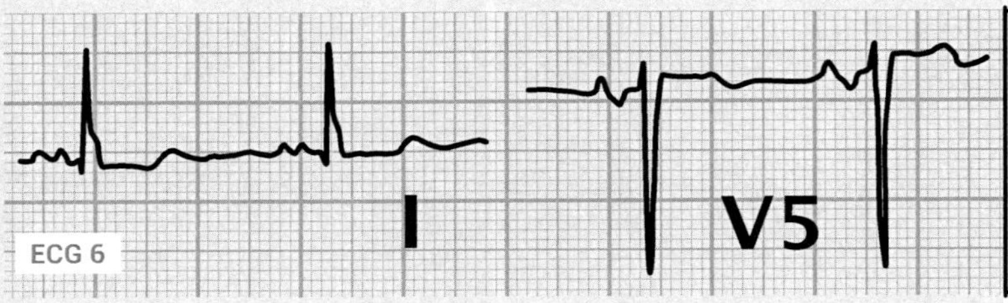

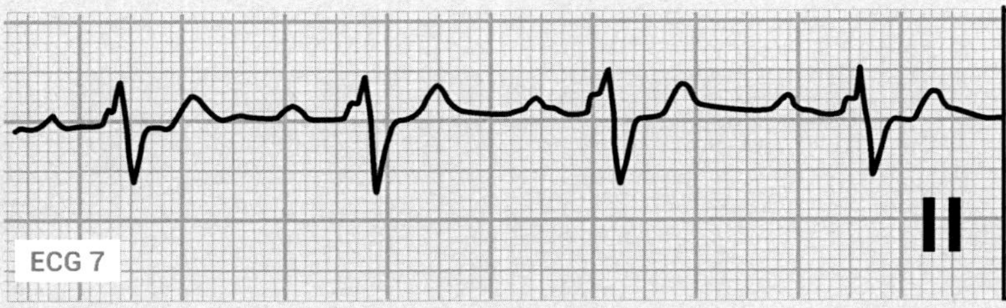

	P mitrale	I° AV block	LGL syndrome	WPW syndrome	Complete bundle branch block	None of the answers provided
ECG 4						
ECG 5						
ECG 6						
ECG 7						

The precordial leads—
what nobody ever tells you

*"The beautiful thing about learning is that nobody
can take it away from you."*

—B.B. King

The precordial leads—what nobody ever tells you

In this chapter you will learn where to put the precordial leads and what they tell you about the heart.

How to place the precordial leads

The precordial leads show the electrical activity of the heart in the horizontal plane. Most commonly, six precordial leads are recorded. The precordial leads are registered in combination with the limb leads. You will learn more about the limb leads in Level 9 of this training.

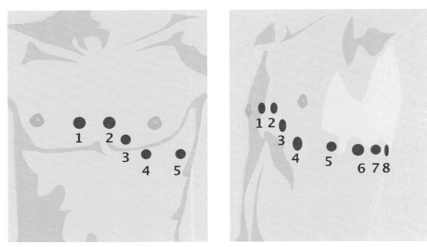

Proper placement of the precordial leads V1 through V6.

The precordial leads are placed at predefined positions on the chest. Here's how to go about it:

1. First, find the second rib and the second intercostal space. Then count down to the fourth intercostal space. Attach V1 in the fourth intercostal space on the right side of the sternum, and attach V2 in the fourth intercostal space on the left side of the sternum.
2. After you've attached V1 and V2, attach V4 at the intersection of the midclavicular line and the fifth intercostal space.
3. Attach V3 exactly halfway in between V2 and V4. From V4 on, we don't need to worry about the intercostal spaces anymore; the subsequent leads are attached at the same horizontal level as V4.
4. V5 is placed in the anterior axillary line (same level as V4).
5. V6 is placed in the midaxillary line (same level as V4).

Occasionally, two additional leads (V7 and V8) are also attached. V7 is located at the posterior axillary line (same level as V4), and V8 is attached at the scapular line (same level as V4).

How to find and count the intercostal spaces correctly

The easiest way to find the fourth intercostal space is to look for the sternal angle. The sternal angle is a little edge in the upper third of the sternum (see image), which can be found in almost any patient. The second rib inserts right next to the sternal angle. Below the second rib is the second intercostal space. Then you just count down to the fourth and fifth intercostal spaces, respectively.

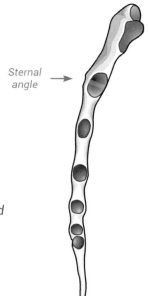
Sternal angle →

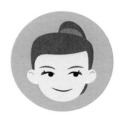
Try to find the second rib on yourself using this approach, and you'll see that it's easy. Then count the intercostal spaces.

What anatomical regions are depicted by what leads?

Each precordial lead depicts a certain region of the heart. Some leads even depict more than one region. Let's say you see ST elevations on the ECG—a sign of myocardial infarction. Just by looking at the affected leads, you'll be able to tell where the infarction is located.

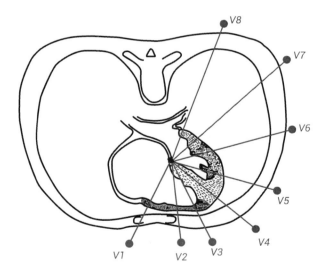

The changes in the right ventricular myocardium can be seen in leads V1, V2, and V3.

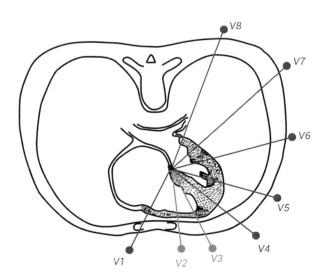

But changes in the basal septum also can be detected in these leads, although usually only in V2 and V3.

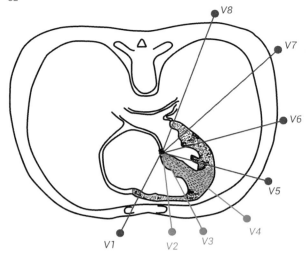

V2, V3, V4: anterior wall of the LV
If changes can be seen in V2, V3, and V4,
then the anterior wall of the left ventricle
(and the septum) are affected.

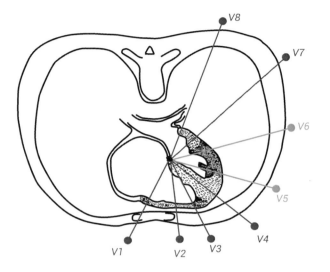

V5, V6: lateral wall of the LV
V5 and V6 show the lateral wall of
the left ventricle.

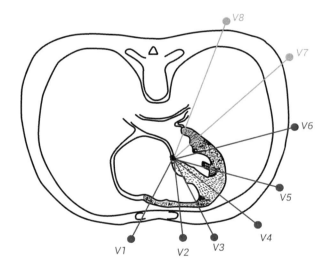

V7, V8: posterior wall
V7 and V8 depict the posterior
wall of the left ventricle.

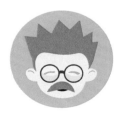

Changes that are seen in the anterior AND the lateral walls are called
anterolateral. *Changes that are seen in the lateral and posterior walls
are called* **posterolateral**. *Changes that are seen in the anterior wall
and the septum are called* **anteroseptal**.

The normal pattern

Each precordial lead has a typical ECG pattern. Try to remember this picture of normal chest leads:

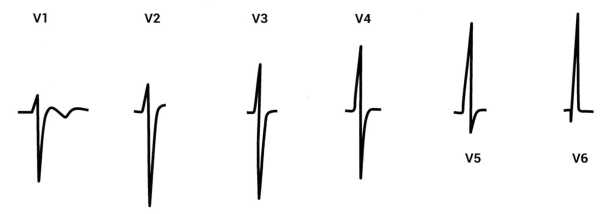

The R/S ratio ("R to S ratio")

As the name implies, the R/S ratio compares the size of the R wave to the size of the S wave in each lead. Let's look at four examples. Please complete the calculations for examples 3 and 4 (answers are at the end of the chapter).

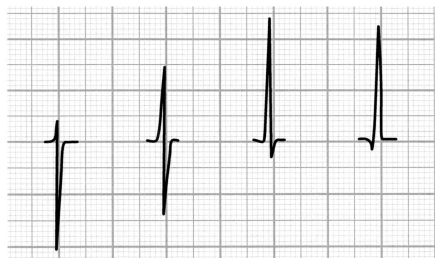

	Example 1	Example 2	Example 3	Example 4
R (mV)	0.4	1.4		
S (mV)	2.0	1.4		
R/S	0.4/2.0 = 1/5 = 0.2	1.4/1.4 = 1		

[Solution at end of chapter]

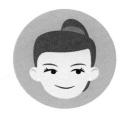

A lot of doctors neglect the R to S ratio. But you shouldn't!

So why is the R/S ratio important?

There are two very important laws that apply under normal circumstances (i.e., when the muscle mass of the left ventricle exceeds that of the right ventricle). Law number 1 says:

Leads with an R/S ratio <1 correspond to the right ventricle

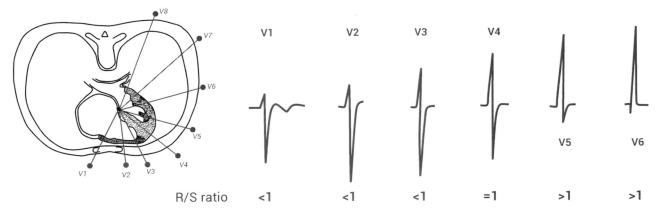

Leads with an R/S ratio >1 correspond to the left ventricle

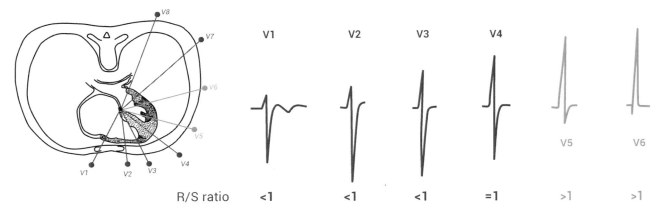

Leads with an R/S ratio of =1 correspond to the transitional zone between right and left ventricle
The transitional zone usually occurs at leads V3 or V4.

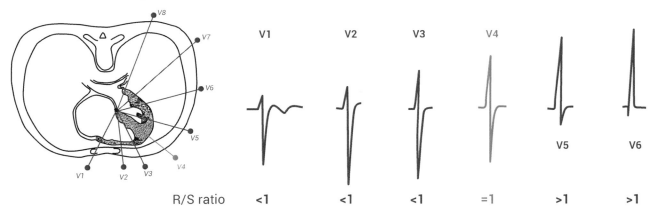

And law number 2 says:

Under normal circumstances, the R/S ratio increases as you go from right to left

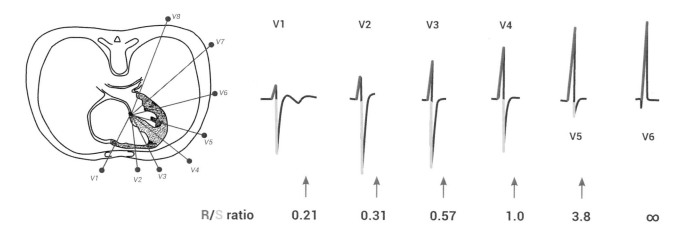

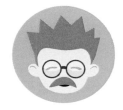

It's also important to note that the amplitude of the initial R wave increases as we go from V1 over to the left ventricle.

When the transitional zone is off

As you learned above, the transitional zone (the dotted line separating right from left ventricle) usually occurs at V3 or V4, as depicted in this image:

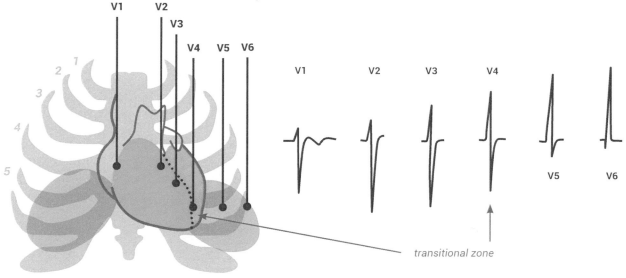

But not every heart is the same. Sometimes, the heart is "rotated" in a clockwise or counterclockwise fashion along its longitudinal axis (going from the apex to the base of the heart).

When the heart is rotated in a clockwise fashion, the transitional zone shifts toward V5 or V6:

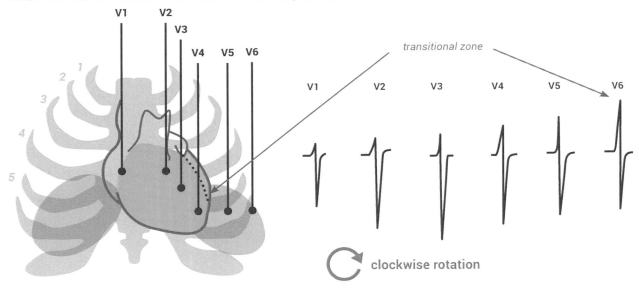

And when the heart is rotated in a counterclockwise fashion, the transitional zone occurs at V1 or V2:

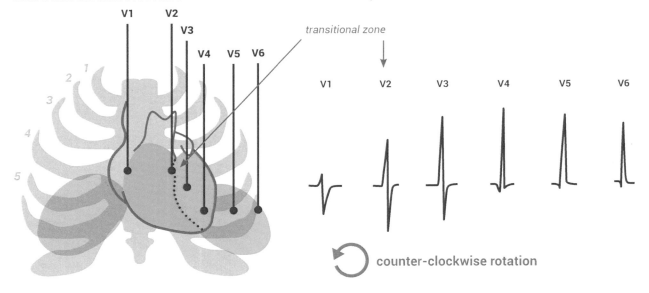

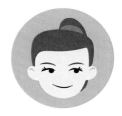 *You'll need to be able to tell whether a precordial lead depicts the right or the left ventricle. Knowledge about rotation is therefore critical.*

Answers to R/S ratio calculations:

	Example 1	Example 2	Example 3	Example 4
R (mV)	0.4	1.4	2.4	2.3
S (mV)	2.0	1.4	0.3	0
R/S	0.4/2.0 = 1/5 = 0.2	1.4/1.4 = 1	8.0	∞

Level 4

QUIZ SECTION

Now it's time for some exercises. They will help you to repeat and remember
the most important information covered in this level.

Which leads provide information on the...	V1	V2	V3	V4	V5	V6	V7	V8
Right ventricle								
Upper part of the septum								
Left ventricle								
Anterior wall of the LV								
Lateral wall of the LV								
Posterior wall of the LV								

Which ventricle is represented by these leads under normal circumstances?

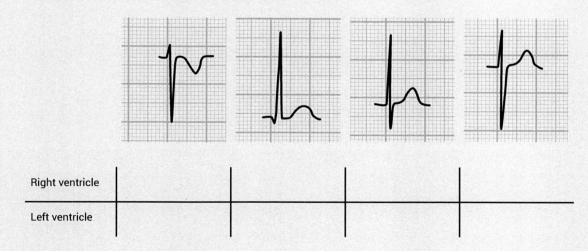

Right ventricle				
Left ventricle				

The chest leads—100% confidence

"Wherever the art of Medicine is loved, there is also a love of Humanity."
—Hippocrates

The chest leads—100% confidence

*In this chapter you'll learn how to recognize abnormal patterns
in the chest leads.*

A normal ECG

It's very important that you remember the normal appearance of the precordial (chest) leads.
So take a look at this example of a normal ECG again:

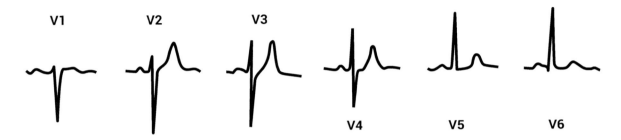

In the right ventricle (V1 and V2), we can usually see small R waves and large S waves in normal individuals. In the left
ventricle (V5 and V6), small Q waves and narrow and tall R waves are usually seen in normal individuals.

Patterns in abnormal ECGs

In abnormal QRS complexes, you'll see a pattern that may be referred to as notching, slurring, an
M shape, or an RSR pattern:

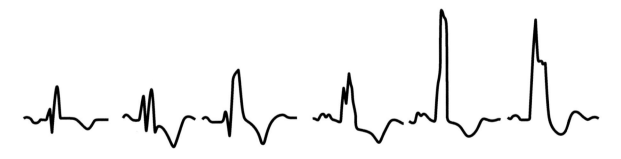

abnormal patterns seen in V1 or V2   *abnormal patterns seen in V5 or V6*

Let's take a closer look:

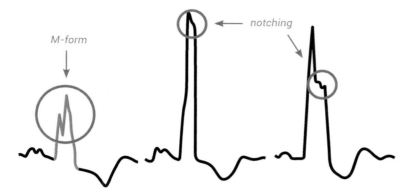

The M pattern is usually quite easy to see. When the delay in depolarization of the ventricles is less obvious, then that's called notching.

These changes in R-wave morphology indicate that depolarization of the ventricles is delayed.

When the QRS duration is between 0.10 and 0.12 seconds, that's called **incomplete bundle branch block**, which causes notching of the QRS complex. Incomplete bundle branch block may be caused by dilatation of the ventricles. It's also referred to as **volume overload**.

In **complete bundle branch block**, conduction through the left or right bundle branch is completely blocked. Depolarization of the ventricles therefore takes longer than normal, and the QRS complex is lengthened to 0.12 seconds or longer.

To find out whether the left or the right bundle branch is affected, we need to look at the chest leads:

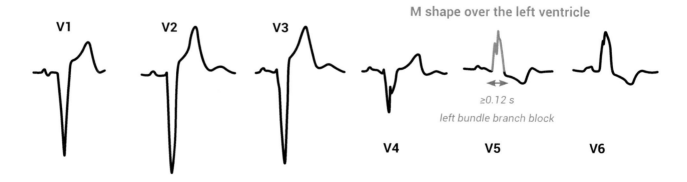

In complete left bundle branch block (LBBB), the QRS duration is ≥0.12 seconds and an M pattern (notching) is seen over the left ventricle (V5 or V6).

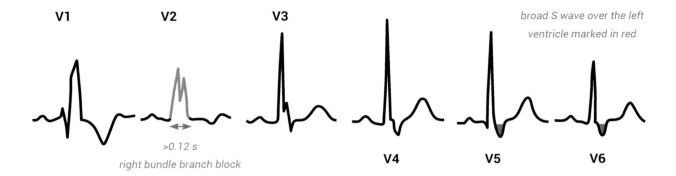

V1 **V2** **V3**

broad S wave over the left
ventricle marked in red

>0.12 s
right bundle branch block

V4 **V5** **V6**

In complete right bundle branch block (RBBB), the QRS duration is ≥0.12 seconds and an M pattern (or notching) is seen over the right ventricle (V1 or V2).

There's one important pathologic condition that could be confused with bundle branch block because QRS duration is also lengthened. You have already learned about this disease in Level 3. Here's an example. Can you spot the problem?

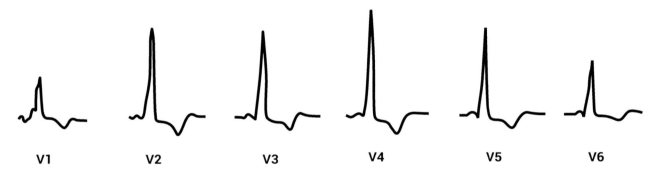

V1 **V2** **V3** **V4** **V5** **V6**

In this example, the QRS duration is lengthened to ≥0.12 seconds and there's notching in lead V1. Is this a case of right bundle branch block?

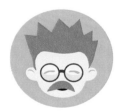

You might have already realized what's wrong with this ECG. There are a few problems: the QRS is lengthened, the PR interval is too short, AND the beginning of the QRS looks kind of funny.

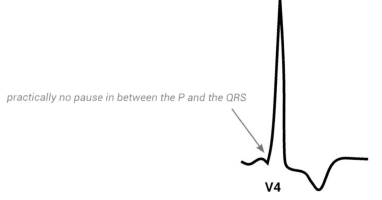

practically no pause in between the P and the QRS

V4

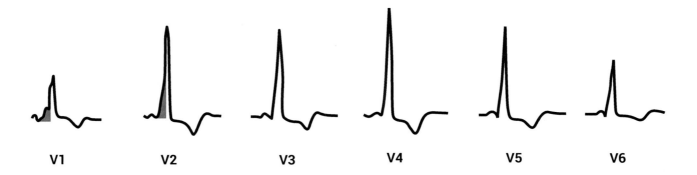

V1   V2   V3   V4   V5   V6

This is a clear case of **WPW syndrome**: the QRS is lengthened, the PR interval is shortened, and a delta wave is present. You'll get the chance to see a lot more examples of this disease in the quizzes.

Sometimes WPW syndrome may look like LBBB with predominant R waves over the left ventricle and predominant S waves over the right ventricle:

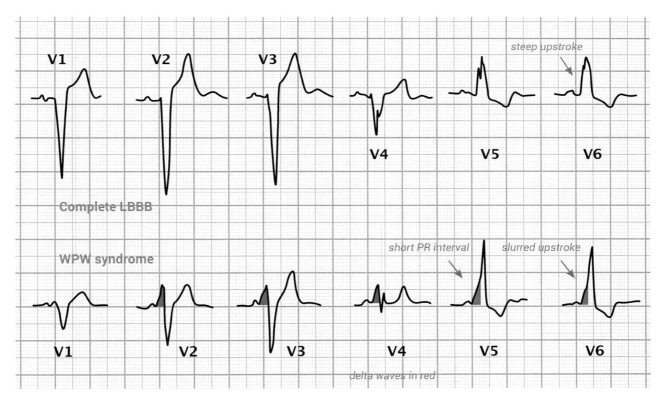

In LBBB, the upstroke of the QRS is steeper than that in WPW syndrome. The short PR interval will also give you a clue into the direction of WPW.

Level 5

QUIZ SECTION

Now it's time for some exercises...

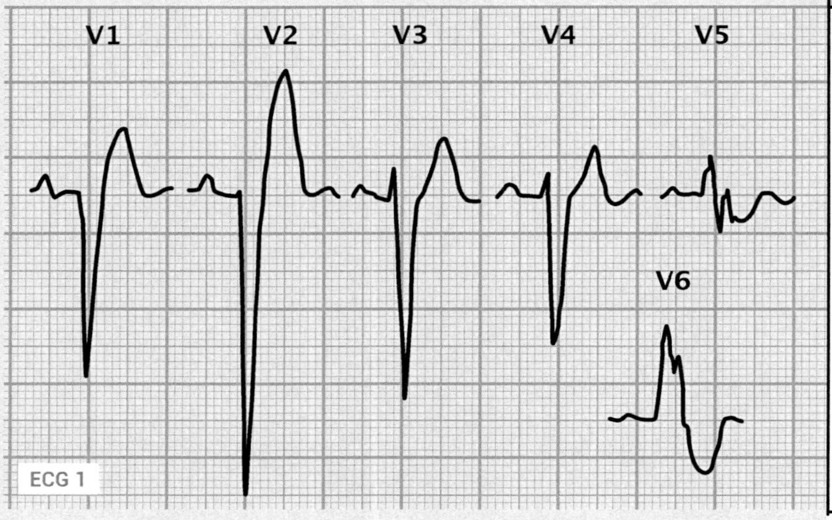

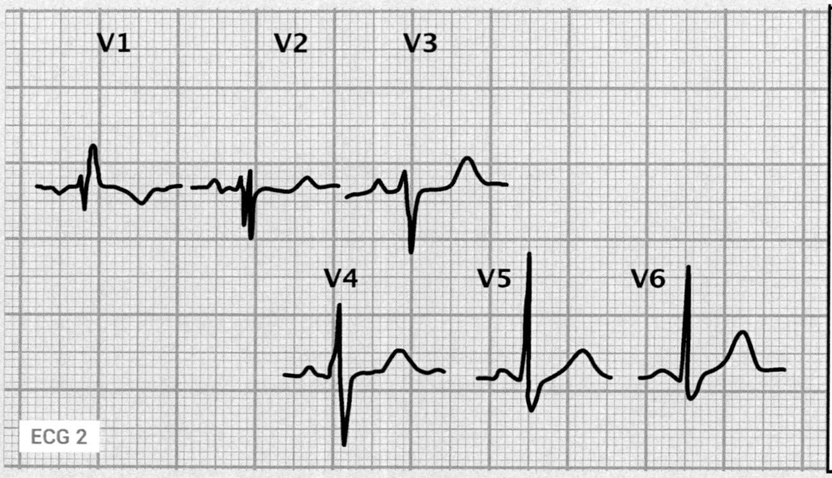

	Diagnosis					Diagnostic criteria				
Complete right bundle branch block	Complete left bundle branch block	Volume overload right ventricle	Volume overload left ventricle	WPW syndrome		Duration of the QRS complex	(V1) QRS shape	(V6) QRS shape	Duration of the PR interval	Delta wave in leads:

ECG 1

V1　V2　V3　V4　V5　V6

ECG 2

V1　V2　V3　V4　V5　V6

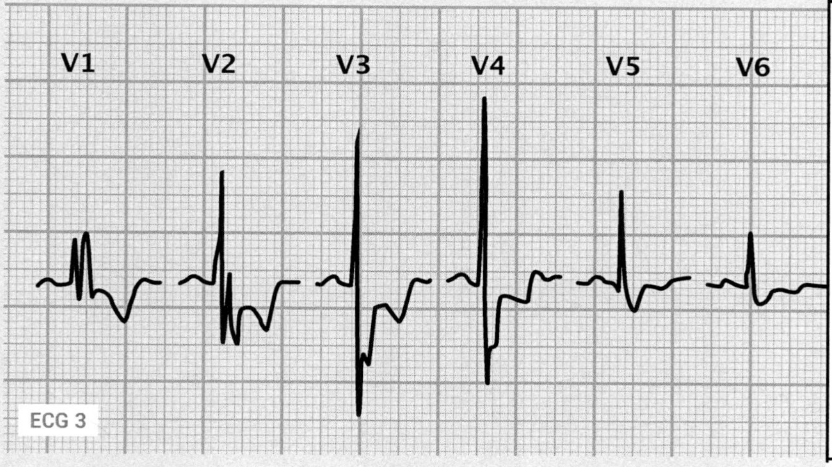

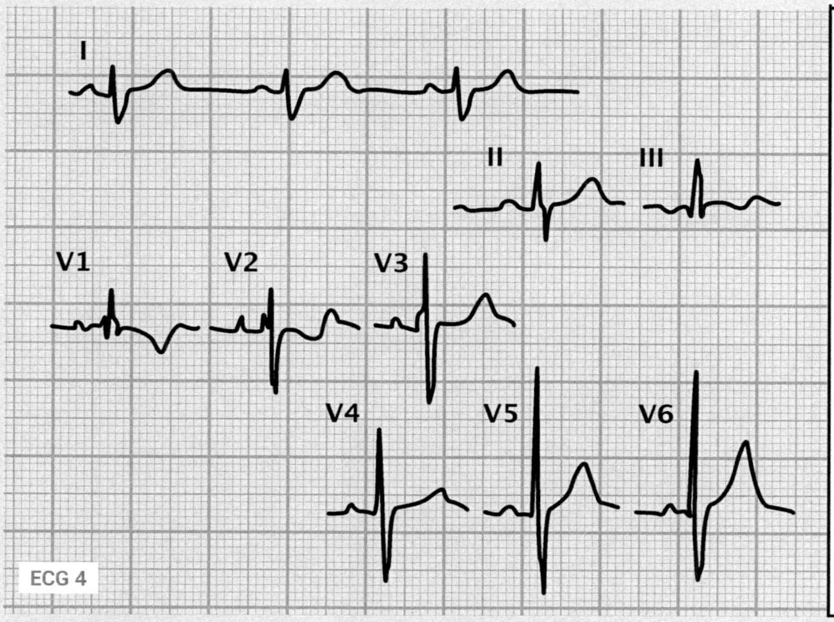

	Diagnosis					Diagnostic criteria				
Complete right bundle branch block	Complete left bundle branch block	Volume overload right ventricle	Volume overload left ventricle	WPW syndrome		Duration of the QRS complex	(V1) QRS shape	(V6) QRS shape	Duration of the PR interval	Delta wave in leads:

V1　V2　V3　V4　V5　V6

ECG 3

I

II　III

V1　V2　V3

V4　V5　V6

ECG 4

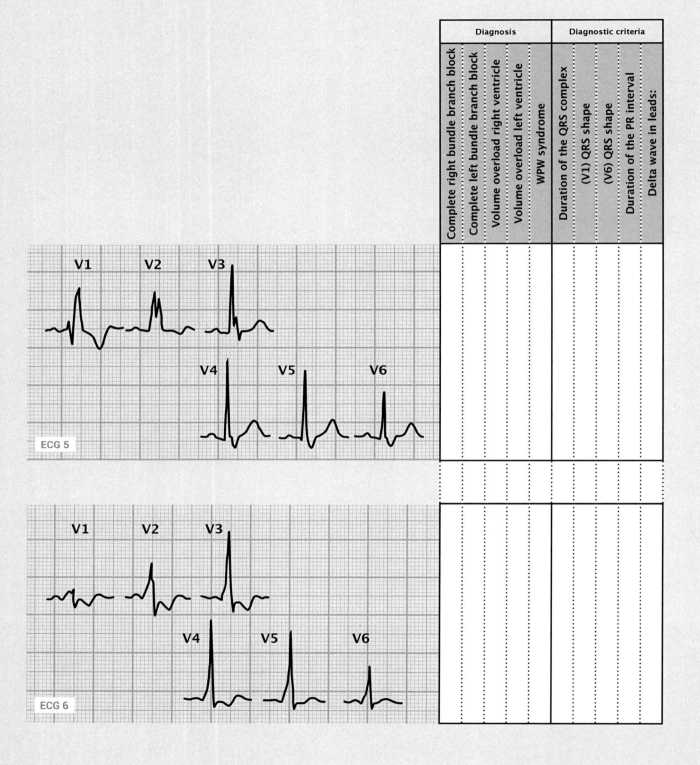

	Diagnosis					Diagnostic criteria				
Complete right bundle branch block	Complete left bundle branch block	Volume overload right ventricle	Volume overload left ventricle	WPW syndrome		Duration of the QRS complex	(V1) QRS shape	(V6) QRS shape	Duration of the PR interval	Delta wave in leads:

ECG 5

ECG 6

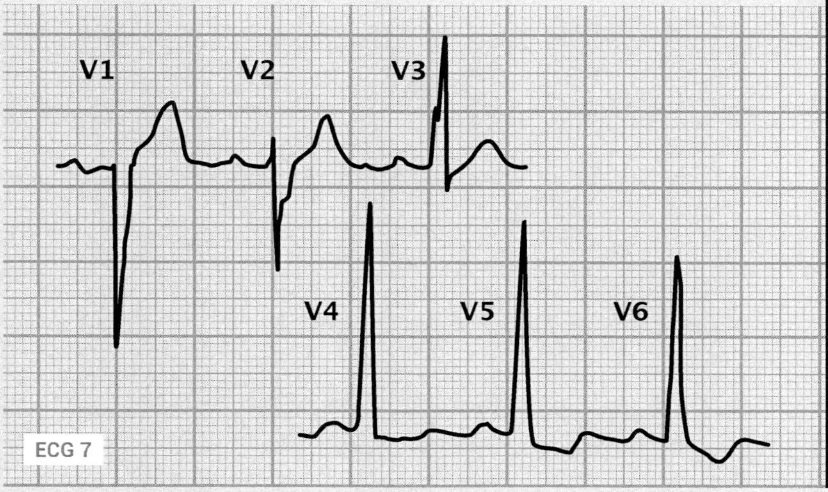

ECG 7

	Diagnosis					Diagnostic criteria				
Complete right bundle branch block	Complete left bundle branch block	Volume overload right ventricle	Volume overload left ventricle	WPW syndrome		Duration of the QRS complex	(V1) QRS shape	(V6) QRS shape	Duration of the PR interval	Delta wave in leads:

What you really need to know about ventricular hypertrophy

"For the things we have to learn before we can do them, we learn by doing them."

—Aristotle

What you really need to know about ventricular hypertrophy

The ECG is an important tool for the identification of ventricular hypertrophy. In this chapter, you'll learn what to look for.

Key concepts

We learned in Level 4 that R waves increase as we go from right (V1) to left (V6). The size of the R wave is a reflection of the myocardial mass underneath the lead. That's why the R waves over the thin-walled right ventricle (V1 and V2) are smaller than the R waves over the muscular left ventricle (V5 and V6).

The waves of the ECG are a product of electrical depolarization. If depolarization moves toward a lead, the respective segment of the ECG wave will be positive. If depolarization moves away from the lead, the deflection will be negative.

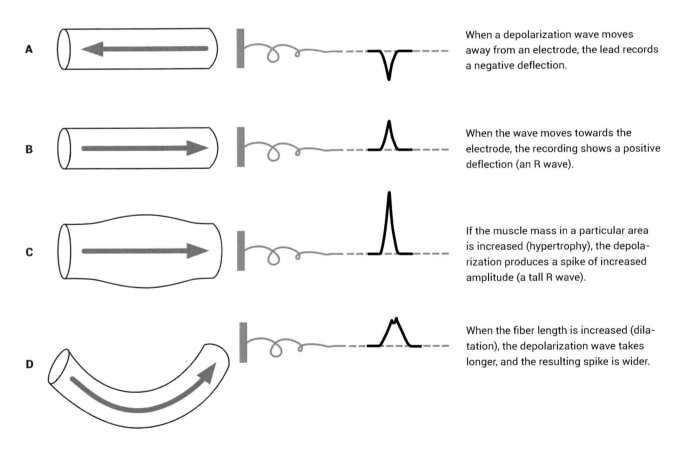

A — When a depolarization wave moves away from an electrode, the lead records a negative deflection.

B — When the wave moves towards the electrode, the recording shows a positive deflection (an R wave).

C — If the muscle mass in a particular area is increased (hypertrophy), the depolarization produces a spike of increased amplitude (a tall R wave).

D — When the fiber length is increased (dilatation), the depolarization wave takes longer, and the resulting spike is wider.

It follows that a strong electrical vector that points in the direction of V5 and V6 produces a large R wave in V5 or V6 and a deep S wave in the opposite leads V1 and V2. In other words, the S wave in V1 and V2 is more or less a mirror image of the R wave in V5 and V6.

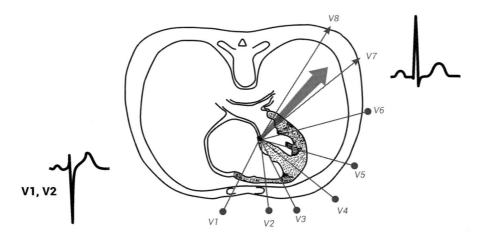

V1, V2

So remember these two important points:

- The higher the R wave over the left ventricle, the larger the muscular mass of the left ventricle (a direct sign of left ventricular hypertrophy).
- The deeper the S wave over the right ventricle, the larger the muscular mass of the left ventricle (an indirect sign of left ventricular hypertrophy).

The Sokolow index

Under normal circumstances the left ventricle has a higher muscular mass than the right ventricle. To assess whether (abnormal) left ventricular hypertrophy is present, the Sokolow index can be used. It basically takes the preceding two statements and turns them into numbers. Here is how it's done:

1. Take the R wave (mV) in V5 or V6 (whichever one is taller).
2. Add the S wave (mV) in V1 or V2 (whichever one is deeper).
3. If the resulting number is more than 3.5 mV, left ventricular hypertrophy is probably present.

Sometimes the R wave in a left ventricular lead alone exceeds 2.5 mV; this can also be interpreted as a sign of left ventricular hypertrophy.

The following example illustrates how to use the Sokolow index:

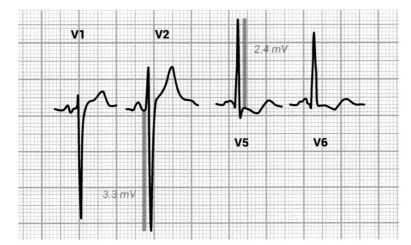

Use the R in V5 because it's taller than the R in V6. The amplitude of that R wave is 2.4 mV. Then measure the S in V2 because it's deeper than the S in V1. That S wave is 3.3 mV. Then add up those numbers: 2.4 + 3.3 = 5.7 mV. Since 5.7 is larger than 3.5, left ventricular hypertrophy is probably present.

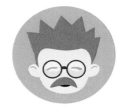

However, this technique should be used with caution. False-positive and false-negative results may occur. Also, this method is not suitable for patients younger than 35 years. A lot of people in this age group will exceed the threshold of 3.5 mV without having left ventricular hypertrophy (which means high rates of false positives!).

Now, let's turn to right ventricular hypertrophy...

The ECG can also be used to assess right ventricular hypertrophy. However, all too often, clinicians forget about it—probably because it's just a little bit trickier than the assessment of left ventricular hypertrophy.

There are a couple of ECG findings that can be used for the assessment of right ventricular hypertrophy. Here are the ones that we find most useful—we call them our **RSS criteria**:

- **Criteria #1:** Look at the **R** wave in V1; present if it's ≥0.5 mV
- **Criteria #2:** Look at the **S** wave in relation to the R wave in V1; present if the R/S ratio in V1 is ≥1
- **Criteria #3:** Look at the **S** wave in V5: present if it's ≥0.5 mV

If two of the three criteria are present, right ventricular hypertrophy is probably present. If right-axis deviation (taught in Level 11) or an incomplete right bundle branch block is also present, the likelihood of right ventricular hypertrophy increases even further.

Here's an example:

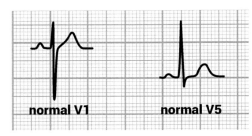

normal patient

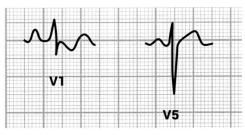

RRS right ventricular hypertrophy
#1: R (V1) = 0.6 mV ⟶ present
#2: R/S (V1) = 0.6/0.4 = 1.5 ⟶ present
#3: S (V5) = 1.3 mV ⟶ present

In this example, all RSS criteria are present. So right ventricular hypertrophy is probably present.

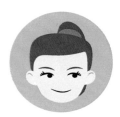

Note that this suspicion always has to be confirmed with echocardiography.

Level 6

QUIZ SECTION

Use the above method to complete the following examples. Fill in your measurements (R waves, S waves, R/S ratios) on the lines below the leads. You don't need to mark the measurements below every lead—just the ones that are relevant. It should be quite obvious from what we've discussed in this level what the relevant leads are. After you've performed the measurements, choose from the four possible diagnoses given on the right side of each example. Use the method taught in Level 4 for the assessment of rotation.

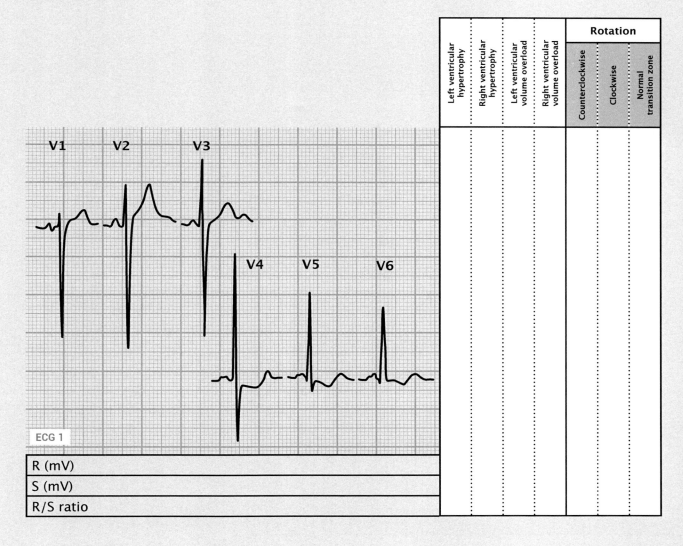

	Left ventricular hypertrophy	Right ventricular hypertrophy	Left ventricular volume overload	Right ventricular volume overload	Rotation		
					Counterclockwise	Clockwise	Normal transition zone
R (mV)							
S (mV)							
R/S ratio							

ECG 1

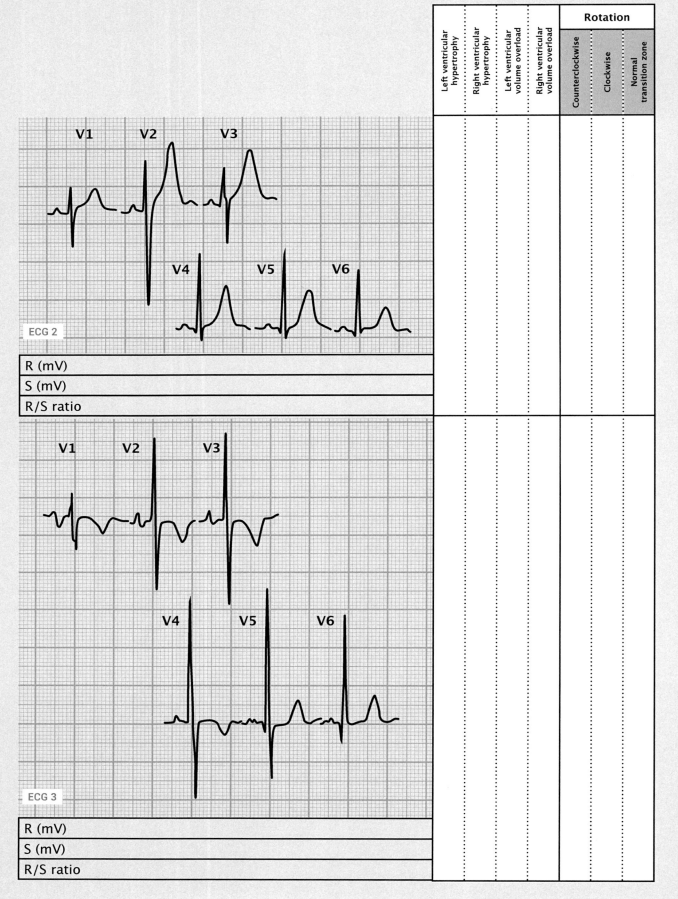

	Left ventricular hypertrophy	Right ventricular hypertrophy	Left ventricular volume overload	Right ventricular volume overload	Rotation		
					Counterclockwise	Clockwise	Normal transition zone

ECG 2

R (mV)	
S (mV)	
R/S ratio	

ECG 3

R (mV)	
S (mV)	
R/S ratio	

	Left ventricular hypertrophy	Right ventricular hypertrophy	Left ventricular volume overload	Right ventricular volume overload	Rotation		
					Counterclockwise	Clockwise	Normal transition zone

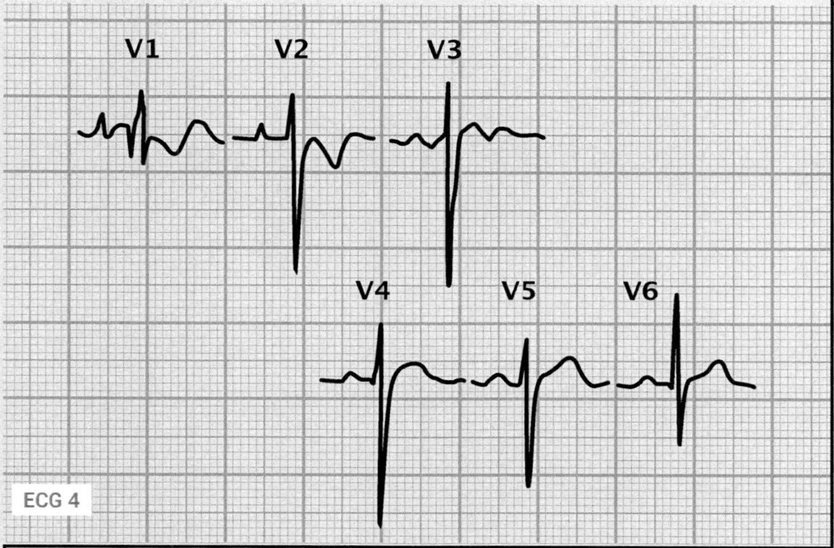

ECG 4

R (mV)							
S (mV)							
R/S ratio							

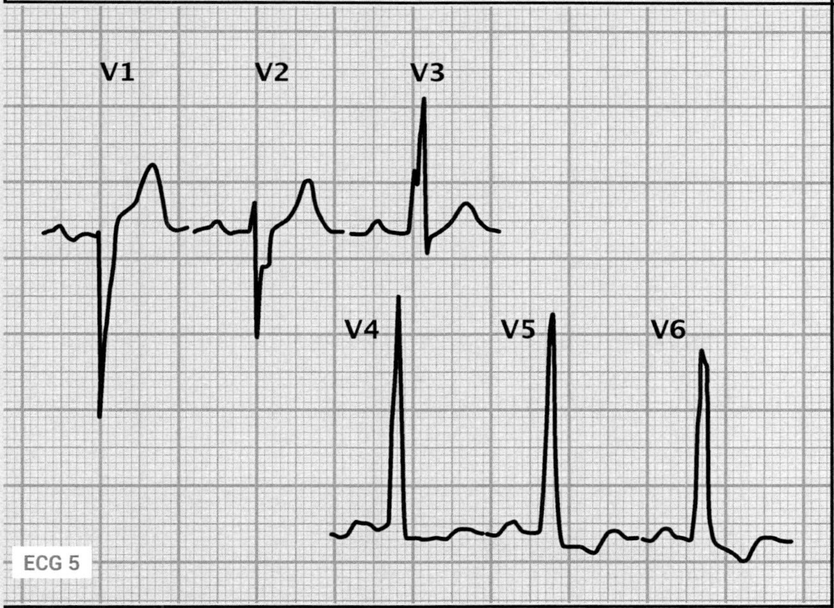

ECG 5

R (mV)							
S (mV)							
R/S ratio							

56

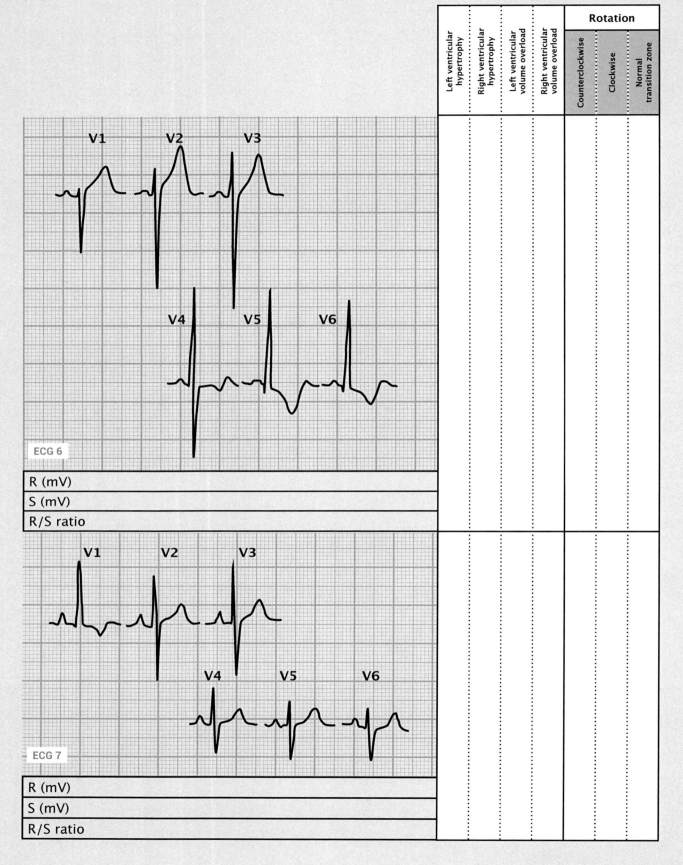

	Left ventricular hypertrophy	Right ventricular hypertrophy	Left ventricular volume overload	Right ventricular volume overload	Rotation		
					Counterclockwise	Clockwise	Normal transition zone

ECG 6

R (mV)							
S (mV)							
R/S ratio							

ECG 7

R (mV)							
S (mV)							
R/S ratio							

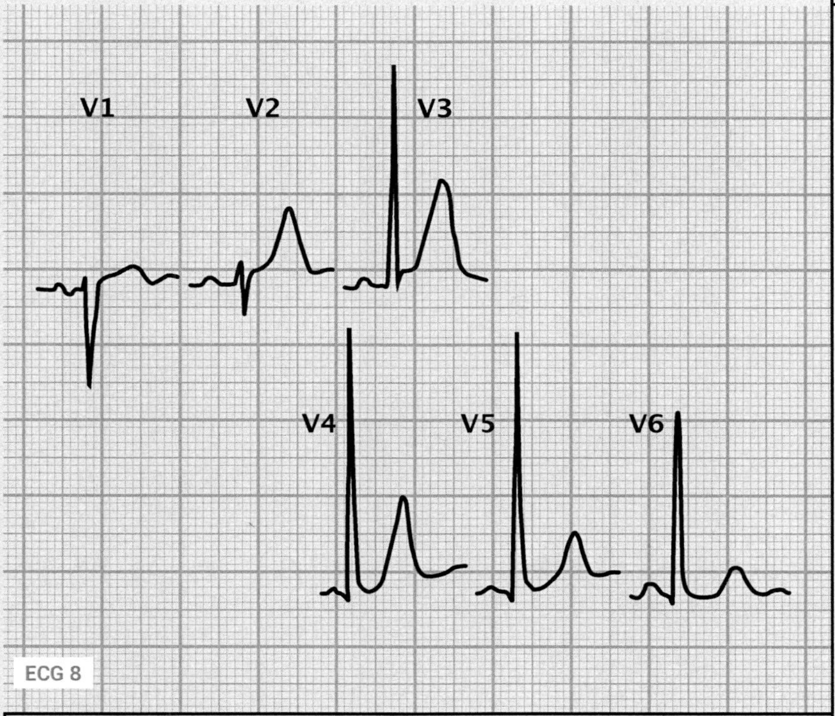

ECG 8

	Left ventricular hypertrophy	Right ventricular hypertrophy	Left ventricular volume overload	Right ventricular volume overload	Rotation		
					Counterclockwise	Clockwise	Normal transition zone
R (mV)							
S (mV)							
R/S ratio							

ST depression and T negativity—
a simple approach

*"Teaching is only demonstrating that it is possible.
Learning is making it possible for yourself."*
—Paulo Coelho

ST depression and T negativity—
a simple approach

ST depression and T-wave negativity are commonly associated with debilitating and potentially life-threatening diseases. Every ECG student should be able to recognize and interpret them. So pay close attention.

Key concepts

Let's start off with two simple principles:

Principle #1:

The ST segment is normally located at the level of the isoelectric line.

By definition, the isoelectric line is located at the level of the ECG curve that comes after the T wave, before the next P wave.

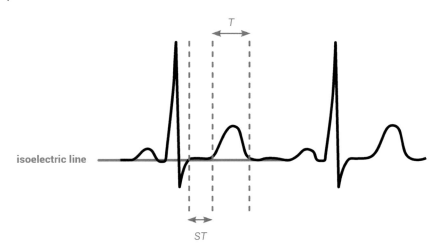

isoelectric line

Principle #2:

Except for V1, the T wave is normally positive.

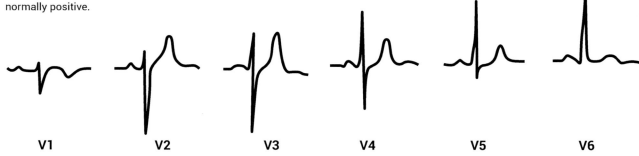

V1　　　　**V2**　　　　**V3**　　　　**V4**　　　　**V5**　　　　**V6**

Once you recognize the presence of ST depressions or T-wave inversions, you should look at two things:

1. Their location (which leads are affected).

2. Their shape.

In Level 4, you learned what leads depict which parts of the ventricle. So if ST depression is present in V5 and V6, for example, you know that the lateral wall is the problem.

The different forms of ST depressions

In our experience, you can tell a lot about the underlying diseases if you know how they change the appearance of the ST segment. Here are some examples:

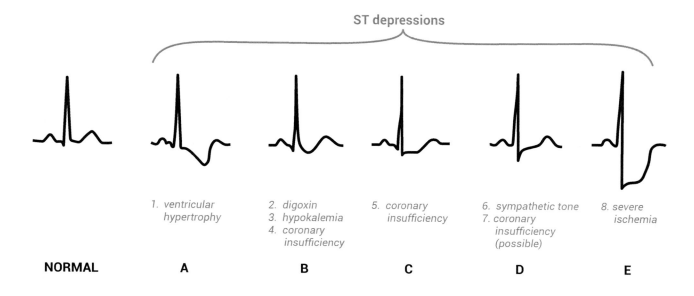

- **Example A:** A descending ST depression is usually associated with ventricular hypertrophy.

- **Examples B, C and D:** These are only relevant over the left ventricle. (One exception to this rule is mirror images of a posterior wall ST elevation myocardial infarction, which will also produce similar ST depressions in V1, V2, and V3. More about that in Level 9.)

- **Example B:** ST depression with a sagging shape—this may be caused by coronary insufficiency (angina), digoxin, or hypokalemia.

- **Example C:** Horizontal ST depression, typically seen in patients with coronary insufficiency (i.e., symptomatic coronary heart disease).

- **Examples B and C:** Commonly seen in patients with exercise-induced angina undergoing stress test.

- **Example D:** Ascending ST depression may be caused by high sympathetic tone, but also by physical activity. During physical activity, ascending ST depressions do not necessarily mean that ischemia is present.

- **Example E:** Deep horizontal ST depressions are often seen in several corresponding leads in the setting of severe ischemia.

Patterns of negative T waves (also known as T-wave inversions)

Here are the most important patterns of inverted T waves:

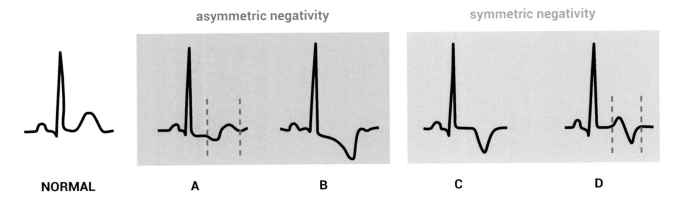

NORMAL   A   B   C   D

Different patterns of T-wave inversions.

On the far left side, you can see a normal T wave for comparison. The other four patterns are negative and therefore abnormal. There's an important distinction that you need to make here:

- The T waves in examples A and B are **asymmetric**. They are slowly downward sloping with an abrupt return to the isoelectric line.
- The negative T waves in examples C and D, on the other hand, are **symmetric**.

This distinction is important because these changes frequently occur in two distinct settings with very different implications:

- **Asymmetric T-wave inversion** usually occurs in the setting of ventricular hypertrophy. When the left ventricle is hypertrophic, the inversions are located somewhere between V4 and V6. When the right ventricle is affected, they can be seen somewhere between V1 and V3.
- **Symmetric T-wave inversion** occurs in a setting in which myocardial cells are dying off—usually in the setting of myocardial ischemia or myocarditis.

T-wave inversion can also be **biphasic**, as in example A, in which we see a negative–positive pattern, whereas in example D we see a positive–negative pattern (terminally negative). Terminal negativity of the T wave has a high specificity for coronary artery disease, especially when the terminal part is symmetric. T waves are also abnormal if they are not positive enough. With predominant R waves, T waves should be at least 1/8 the size of the R wave. T waves may also be abnormal if they are flat or even horizontal.

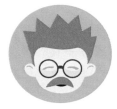

*In right and left **bundle branch block**, repolarization is also impaired. Therefore, we can see negative T waves and ST depressions in leads V1 to V3 in right bundle branch block and in V4 to V6 in left bundle branch block. Two other common problems associated with negative T waves and ST depressions are **premature ventricular beats** and **Wolff-Parkinson-White syndrome**.*

QUIZ SECTION

In the following exercises, please describe the pattern of ST-segment changes (e.g., horizontal, descending, etc.) as well as T-wave changes (e.g., symmetric, asymmetric, biphasic, etc.) and decide what the underlying diagnosis could be.

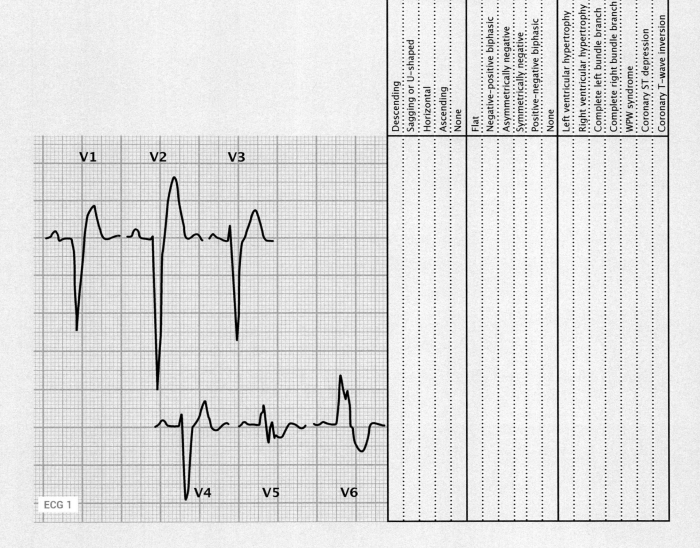

ECG 1

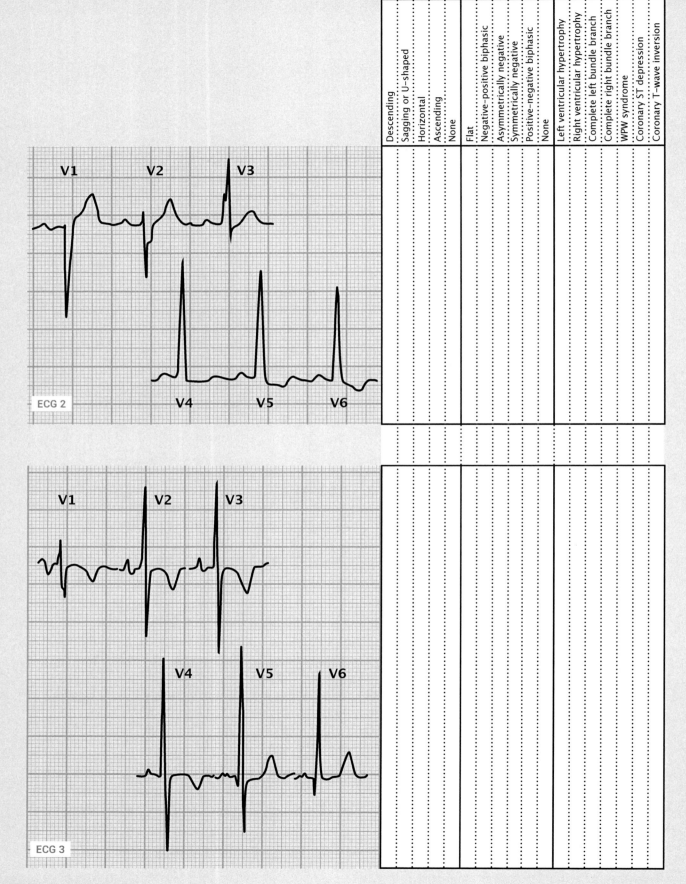

ST depression					T negativity						Diagnosis						
Descending	Sagging or U-shaped	Horizontal	Ascending	None	Flat	Negative–positive biphasic	Asymmetrically negative	Symmetrically negative	Positive–negative biphasic	None	Left ventricular hypertrophy	Right ventricular hypertrophy	Complete left bundle branch	Complete right bundle branch	WPW syndrome	Coronary ST depression	Coronary T-wave inversion
:	:	:	:	:	:	:	:	:	:	:	:	:	:	:	:	:	:

ST depression					T negativity						Diagnosis						
Descending	Sagging or U-shaped	Horizontal	Ascending	None	Flat	Negative–positive biphasic	Asymmetrically negative	Symmetrically negative	Positive–negative biphasic	None	Left ventricular hypertrophy	Right ventricular hypertrophy	Complete left bundle branch	Complete right bundle branch	WPW syndrome	Coronary ST depression	Coronary T-wave inversion

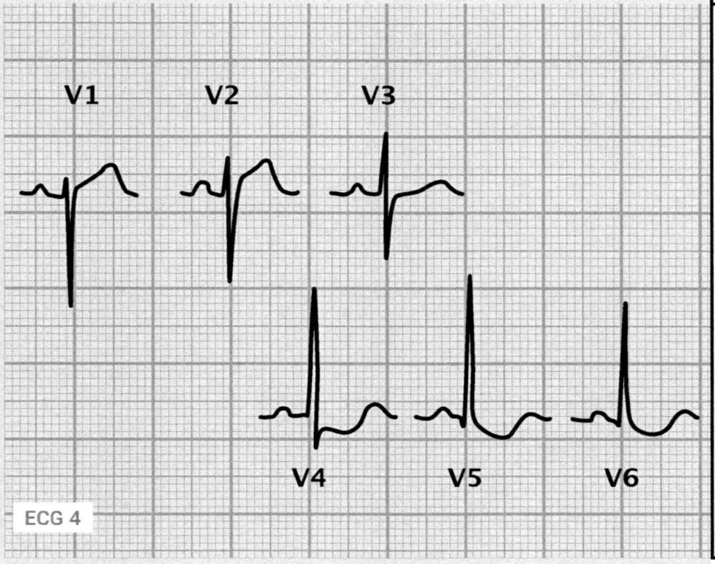

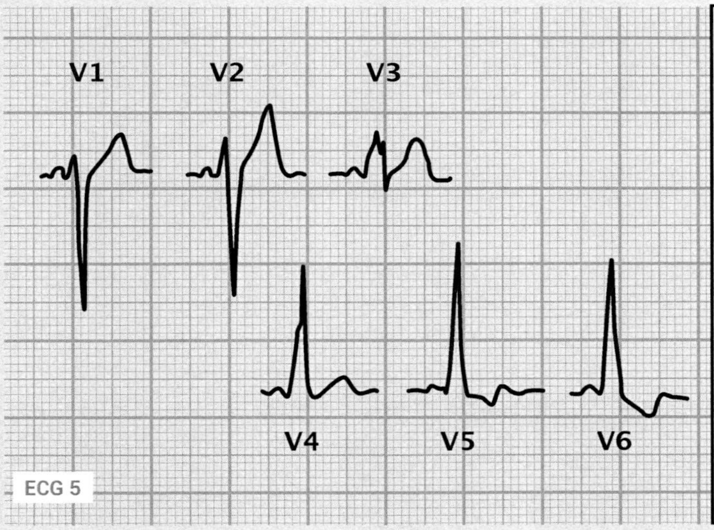

ECG 4

ECG 5

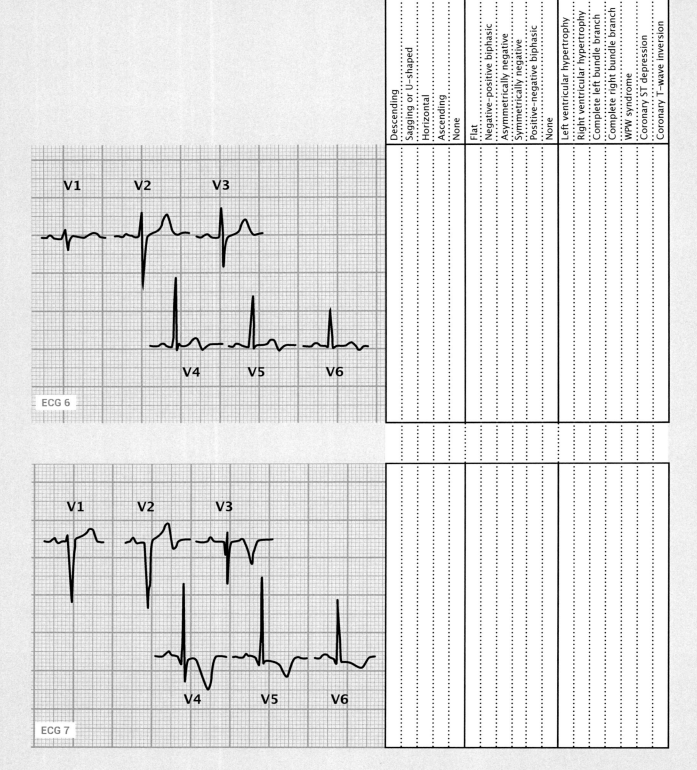

	ST depression					T negativity						Diagnosis						
	Descending	Sagging or U-shaped	Horizontal	Ascending	None	Flat	Negative–positive biphasic	Asymmetrically negative	Symmetrically negative	Positive–negative biphasic	None	Left ventricular hypertrophy	Right ventricular hypertrophy	Complete left bundle branch	Complete right bundle branch	WPW syndrome	Coronary ST depression	Coronary T-wave inversion
ECG 6																		
ECG 7																		

What everybody ought to know about myocardial infarction and the QRS complex

"The only thing better than education is more education."

—Agnes E. Benedict

What everybody ought to know about myocardial infarction and the QRS complex

In this chapter, you will learn how myocardial infarction affects the appearance of the QRS complex.

Drowning in negativity

There's one big idea that you have to keep in mind to remember what myocardial infarction does to the QRS complex. And the big idea is this: **drowning in negativity.**

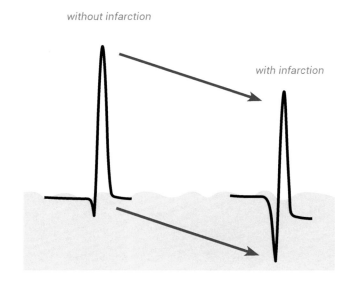

without infarction

with infarction

Drowning means that certain parts of the QRS become negative (Q waves) while other parts will decrease in size (R waves). In other words, one or more of the following things can happen:

- A preexisting **R wave decreases** in size
- A preexisting **Q wave gets deeper**
- A **new Q wave** develops

The resulting pattern is highly dependent on the initial form of the QRS complex. As we've said before, if you know what the QRS complex in each lead looks like, you'll also know when something's wrong.

Let's have a look at some examples:

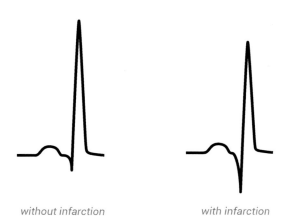

without infarction   *with infarction*

Example A: In this example, there's an initial Q wave even without myocardial infarction. This could be V5 or V6 where we would typically see a small Q wave even in normal patients. When myocardial infarction develops, the Q wave gets much deeper than before—here it's 1/3 the size of the R wave.

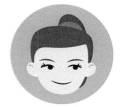

Small Q waves can be present in leads V5, V6, I, aVL, II, and III of healthy patients.

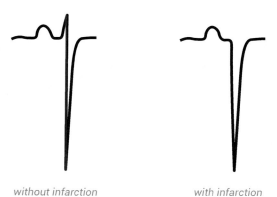

without infarction   with infarction

Example B: Here we have a small initial R wave. This is the typical appearance of leads V1 or V2. When myocardial infarction develops, the R gets lost and we end up with one deep QS complex.

Example C: In this example, the R wave is already pretty tall (left side, without infarction), while the S is still fairly deep (R/S ratio <1). So this must be an area under leads V2 to V4. In these leads we usually don't see any Q waves. But when myocardial infarction develops, there's a new Q wave at the beginning of the QRS complex—the initial R wave is lost.

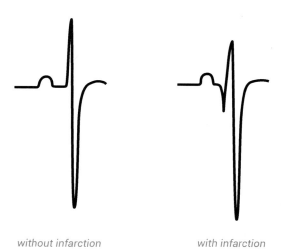

without infarction   with infarction

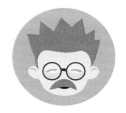

These changes appear over the parts of the ventricle that are affected by myocardial infarction, which makes localization of the affected area fairly easy.

It's useful to know that these changes to the QRS complex can be seen in both acute and old myocardial infarctions. When you observe them in a patient who does not have any symptoms of acute myocardial infarction, this probably means that you are dealing with an old infarct.

Pathologic or not pathologic—that is the question

It can sometimes be tricky to differentiate between normal Q waves and pathologic Q waves. Pathologic Q waves in the setting of myocardial infarction are usually deeper and wider than normal Q waves. The criteria for pathologic Q waves are:

- The depth of the Q wave is ≥1/4 the size of the R wave in the same lead.

or

- The Q-wave duration is >0.04 seconds (1 small box on the ECG paper).

There are a couple of additional criteria, but these are the ones you should remember for now.

One other trick that you can use in the precordial leads is to look at the Q-wave progression in leads V4 to V6. Under normal conditions, the depth of the Q wave increases as we go from V4 (where in most cases there is no Q-wave yet) to V6, as seen in the following example:

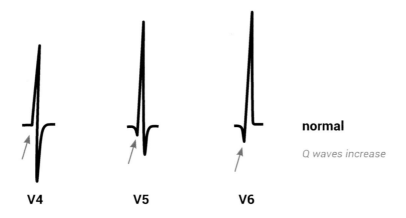

normal

Q waves increase

V4   **V5**   **V6**

However, when there's an infarct in the area of V4 and V5, Q waves will decrease in size as we go from V4 to V6, as seen in the following example:

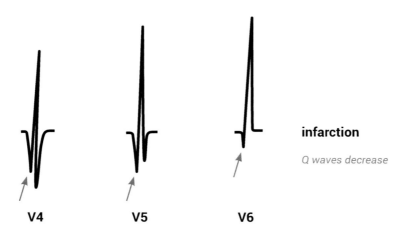

infarction

Q waves decrease

V4   **V5**   **V6**

The following image shows an infarct at the anterolateral region. In this example, there will be pathologic Q waves in V4 and V5 that will be bigger and more pronounced than the small Q wave in lead V6.

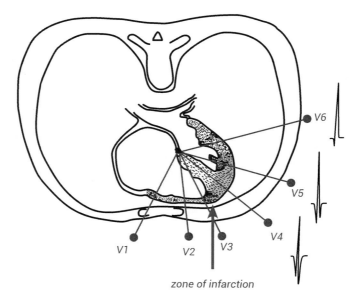

zone of infarction

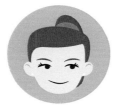

So remember, when Q waves get smaller from V4 to V6, myocardial infarction is probably present in the area around V4.

Now let's have a look at the normal appearance of the precordial leads again:

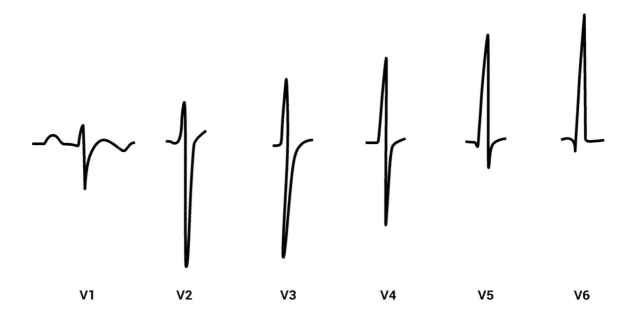

| V1 | V2 | V3 | V4 | V5 | V6 |

Two important tricks for your toolbox

You'll have to learn two important facts that are critical for ECG mastery:

Fact #1 says **leads V1, V2, and V3 usually start with an initial R wave.**

V1 can sometimes come without an initial R wave, but from V2 onward we almost always see it.
In V3 the R wave is usually already pretty big.

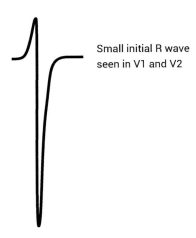

Small initial R wave
seen in V1 and V2

Now take a look at this example:

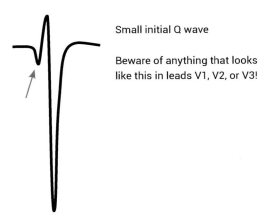

Small initial Q wave

Beware of anything that looks
like this in leads V1, V2, or V3!

This QRS complex also has a small R wave, but there's a small Q wave preceding it. If you see something like this in leads V1, V2, or V3, you should always remember fact #1. Myocardial infarction is very likely in these cases.

Fact #2 says **R-wave amplitudes normally increase as we go from V1 to V6.**

If R-wave amplitude does not increase from V1 to V3 or if R wave amplitude even decreases, we also have to think about the possibility of myocardial infarction in the anterior wall.

Now we'll look at some examples:

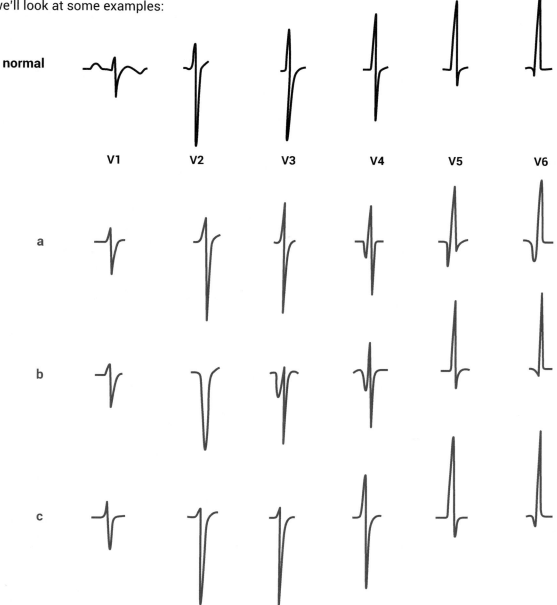

- **Example a:** There are abnormal Q waves in leads V4 to V6. Also, R-wave amplitude decreases from V3 to V4. These are clear signs of myocardial infarction of the anterolateral region (V4 = anterior wall, V5 and V6 = lateral wall).

- **Example b:** The R wave seen in V1 gets completely lost in V2, where we see a large QS complex. Furthermore, pathologic Q waves can be seen in V3 and V4. This is a clear case of an anterior wall myocardial infarction (V2 to V4 = anterior wall).

- **Example c:** Here the signs of myocardial infarction are more subtle than in the previous examples. R-wave amplitude decreases as we go from V1 to V2 and stays the same from V2 to V3. R-wave progression in V4 is normal again. This is probably a case of myocardial infarction of the basal septum (V2 and V3 = basal septum).

Level 8

QUIZ SECTION

Now it's time for some exercises again!

Changes in QRS morphology related to myocardial infarction (pathologic Q wave, QS pattern, reduced initial R wave) can be found in leads									Infarction Localization	Which additional ECG changes can be found? (write them down)
V1	V2	V3	V4	V5	V6	V7	V8	Anteroseptal	
								Anterior wall	
								Lateral wall	
								Anterolateral region	
								Posterior wall	
								Posterolateral region	

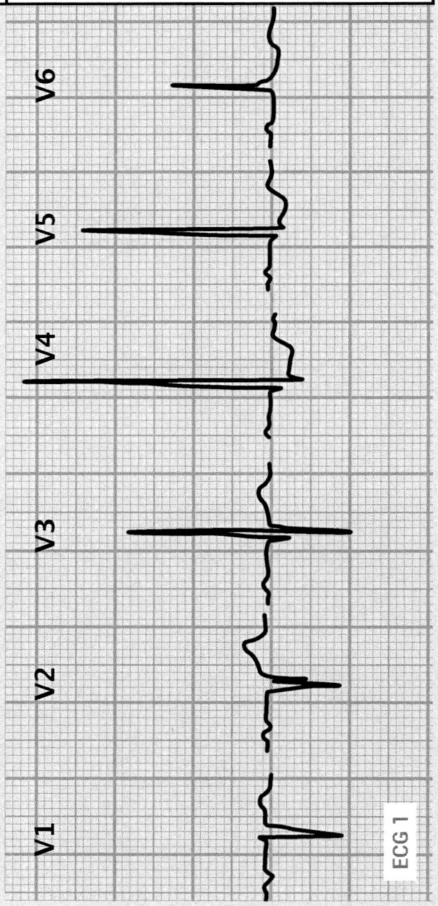

V1 V2 V3 V4 V5 V6

ECG 1

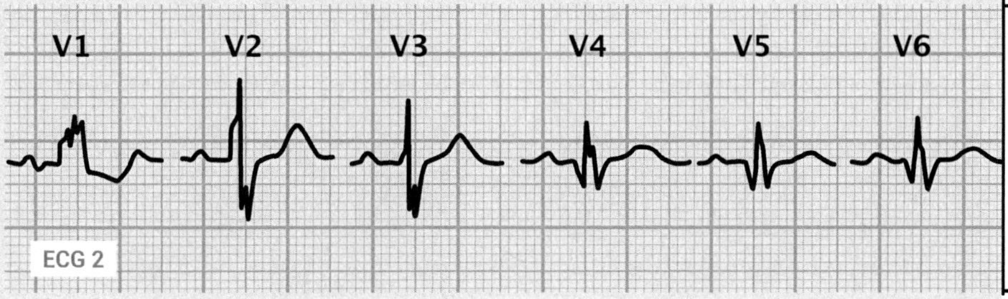

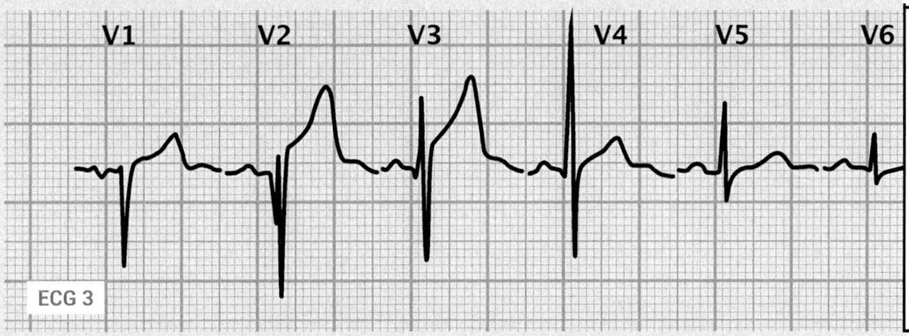

Changes in QRS morphology related to myocardial infarction (pathologic Q wave, QS pattern, reduced initial R wave) can be found in leads									Infarction Localization	Which additional ECG changes can be found? (write them down)
V1	V2	V3	V4	V5	V6	V7	V8		Anteroseptal	
									Anterior wall	
									Lateral wall	
									Anterolateral region	
									Posterior wall	
									Posterolateral region	

ECG 2

ECG 3

Changes in QRS morphology related to myocardial infarction (pathologic Q wave, QS pattern, reduced initial R wave) can be found in leads									Infarction Localization						Which additional ECG changes can be found? (write them down)
V1	V2	V3	V4	V5	V6	V7	V8	Anteroseptal	Anterior wall	Lateral wall	Anterolateral region	Posterior wall	Posterolateral region	
....	....	....	....	....	....	....	....	....	....	....	....	....	....	
....	....	....	....	....	....	....	....	....	....	....	....	....	....	

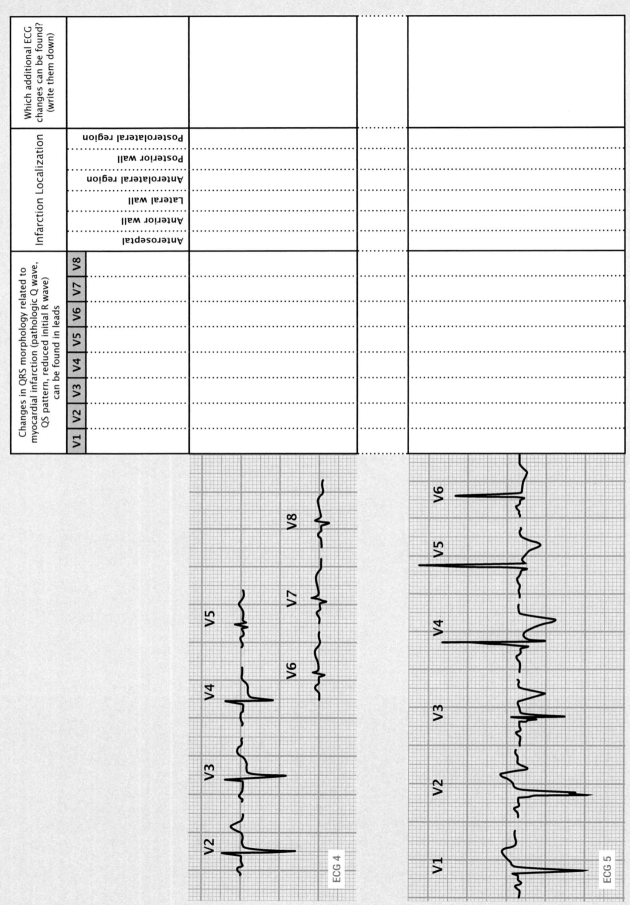

ECG 4

ECG 5

Changes in QRS morphology related to myocardial infarction (pathologic Q wave, QS pattern, reduced initial R wave) can be found in leads									Infarction Localization	Which additional ECG changes can be found? (write them down)
V1	V2	V3	V4	V5	V6	V7	V8		Anteroseptal .... Anterior wall .... Lateral wall .... Anterolateral region .... Posterior wall .... Posterolateral region	

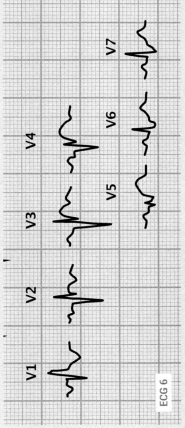

ECG 6

Level 9

Inferior wall myocardial infarction—pearls and pitfalls

"Nothing in life is to be feared, it is only to be understood. Now is the time to understand more, so that we may fear less."
—*Madame Curie*

Inferior wall myocardial infarction—pearls and pitfalls

In the previous chapters, we focused on the precordial leads (chest leads). Learning the ECG works best if you have a thorough understanding of the precordial leads before learning about the limb leads. But now it's time to move on.

The limb leads

The limb leads and the precordial leads view the heart from two different perspectives. The precordial leads more or less show the horizontal plane, whereas the limb leads show the frontal plane.

Limb Leads: Frontal Plane

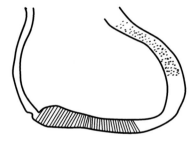

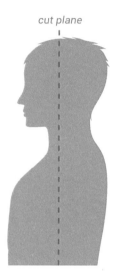

cut plane

Precordial Leads: Horizontal Plane

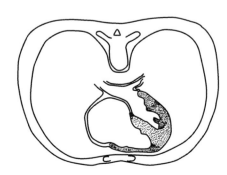

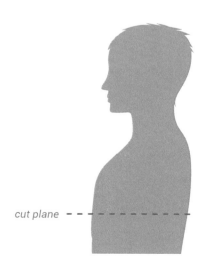

cut plane

The limb leads consist of:

- Three standard leads called **I**, **II**, and **III**
- Three augmented leads called **aVR** (right arm), **aVL** (left arm), and **aVF** (foot)

Four wires are needed to record these leads:

- The **red wire** goes onto the **right arm**.
- The **yellow wire** goes onto the **left arm**.
- The **green wire** goes onto the **left foot**.
- The **black wire** goes onto the **right foot**.

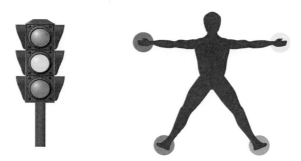

You can remember this sequence by picturing a traffic light with a red light on top, a yellow light in the middle, and a green light on the bottom:

Using these wires, you can now record the limb leads. As we said, these leads look at the electrical activity of the heart in a frontal plane:

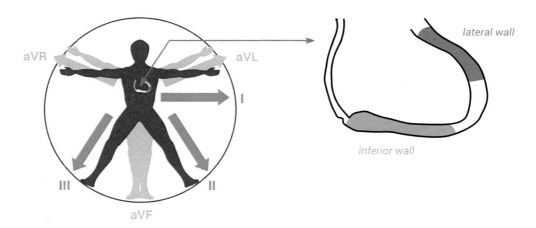

The figure shows that changes of the lateral wall (red area), like myocardial infarction, are depicted by leads I and aVL. Changes in the inferior wall (green area) are depicted by leads II, III, and aVF.

Lead aVR is only occasionally used and you do not need to worry about it for now.

As we already learned, precordial leads V5 and V6 also depict the lateral wall. So we don't absolutely need leads I and aVL to make the diagnosis of problems of the lateral wall like myocardial infarction.

Conversely, the precordial leads don't show the inferior wall—at least not directly. So we need leads II, III, and aVF to evaluate the inferior wall.

Occasionally, leads II, III, and aVF will not detect inferior wall infarction, especially when it's small. That's when a little trick comes in handy.

Looking at mirror images

The direct electrical image of an inferior wall myocardial infarction is visualized in II, III, and aVF. Leads V1, V2, and V3 view the heart from the opposite side and can therefore produce so-called mirror images:

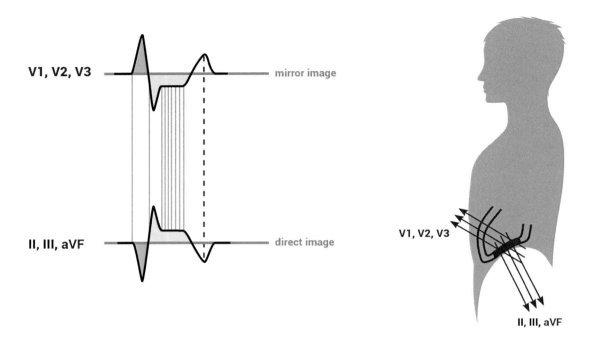

Example of an inferior wall myocardial infarction. Direct changes can be seen in leads II, III, and aVF: deep and broad Q wave, ST elevation, and negative T wave. A mirror image can be seen in leads V1, V2, and V3: broad R wave, ST depression, and positive T wave.

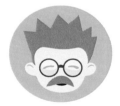

So we have to update our knowledge about the precordial leads. V1, V2, and V3 not only give you information about the right ventricle and the basal septum but also about the inferior wall...in the form of mirror images. A lot of people don't know about this!

Updating our knowledge about the Q-wave criteria

Let's quickly recap the criteria for pathologic Q waves from Level 8. We said that Q waves are pathologic if:

- The depth of the Q wave is ≥1/4 the size of the R wave in the same lead.

or

- The Q wave is >0.04 seconds (1 small box on the ECG paper).

Now there are **two more criteria** for pathologic Q waves:

- Any Q waves in leads V1 to V3 (even if ≤0.04 s) are abnormal.
- In all cases, Q waves have to be present in two contiguous (neighboring) leads. Contiguous leads are I and aVL; II, III, and aVF; and V1 to V6 (e.g., V1 and V2 are contiguous, V3 and V4 are contiguous, etc.).

Q-wave and non−Q-wave infarctions

Not every patient with myocardial infarction develops Q waves. There are Q-wave and non−Q-wave infarctions. The presence and size of Q waves correlate with the extent of myocardial scarring; however, this correlation is far from perfect.

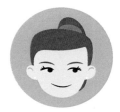

In the olden days, people thought that Q-wave infarctions were transmural (involving the entire thickness of the ventricle) and that non−Q-wave infarctions were only subendocardial. However, pathologic studies have found that this reasoning is flawed and that there were transmural infarctions that did not develop Q waves and subendocardial infarctions that did.

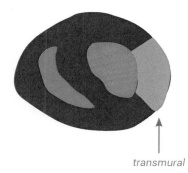

transmural

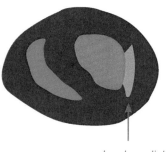

subendocardial

In the next chapter, you will learn how to diagnose myocardial infarction if Q waves are absent.

Please welcome … the ECG cookbook!

Now, it's time to introduce you to our ECG cookbook. The cookbook will provide you with a step-by-step approach for evaluating an actual ECG without missing anything. There are a total of 11 steps in the cookbook. You should be able to complete 5 of them with the knowledge you've acquired so far. We'll add more steps to the cookbook as we progress. We recommend that you make it a habit to go through all the steps of the cookbook when evaluating an ECG. That way you'll make sure not to miss anything, you'll improve the odds of coming up with the right diagnosis, and you'll develop a habit, which will become second nature within a short time.

So without further ado, here's the cookbook....

Question	Answer	Diagnosis
1. Rhythm	[coming later]	[coming later]
2. Heart rate	[coming later]	[coming later]
3. P waves	[coming later]	[coming later]
4. PR interval	a) >0.2 s (if PR interval constant for all beats and each P wave is followed by a QRS complex)	I° AV block
	b) <0.12 s and QRS complex normal	LGL syndrome
	c) <0.12 s and visible delta wave	WPW syndrome
5. QRS axis	[coming later]	[coming later]
6. QRS duration	a) ≥0.12 s (always think of WPW syndrome as a differential)	complete bundle branch block
	b) >0.1 s and <0.12 s with typical bundle branch block appearance (notching)	incomplete bundle branch block
7. Rotation	Rotation is defined according to the heart's transition zone. Normally the transition zone is located at V4, which means that right ventricular myocardium is located at V1–V3 and left ventricular myocardium is at V5–V6.	transition zone at V5–V6: clockwise rotation transition zone at V1–V3: counterclockwise rotation NOTE: don't evaluate rotation in the setting of myocardial infarction, WPW syndrome, or bundle branch block
8. QRS amplitude	a) QRS amplitude <0.5 mV in all standard leads	low voltage
	b) Positive criteria for left ventricular hypertrophy	left ventricular hypertrophy
	c) Positive criteria for right ventricular hypertrophy	right ventricular hypertrophy
9. QRS infarction signs	abnormal Q waves, QS waves, missing R-wave progression	myocardial infarction; localization according to affected leads
10. ST–T segment	[coming later]	[coming later]
11. QT duration, T–U waves	[coming later]	[coming later]

Level 9

QUIZ SECTION

And now it's time for some exercises using our cookbook.

PR	I° AV block		
	WPW syndrome		
	LGL syndrome		
QRS duration	Complete RBBB		
	Complete LBBB		
	Dilated right ventricle		
	Dilated left ventricle		
Rotation	Normal transition zone		
	Clockwise rotation		
	Counterclockwise rotation		
Hypertrophy	Right ventricular hypertrophy		
	Left ventricular hypertrophy		
Infarction	Anteroseptal region		
	Anterior wall		
	Anterolateral region		
	Lateral region		
	Posterolateral region		
	Posterior wall		
	Inferior wall		

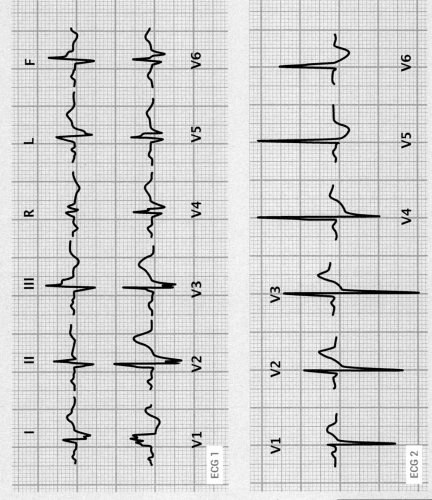

ECG 1

ECG 2

Infarction	Inferior wall		
	Posterior wall		
	Posterolateral region		
	Lateral region		
	Anterolateral region		
	Anterior wall		
	Anteroseptal region		
Hyper-trophy	Left ventricular hypertrophy		
	Right ventricular hypertrophy		
Rotation	Counterclockwise rotation		
	Clockwise rotation		
	Normal transition zone		
QRS duration	Dilated left ventricle		
	Dilated right ventricle		
	Complete LBBB		
	Complete RBBB		
PR	LGL-syndrome		
	WPW-syndrome		
	I° AV block		

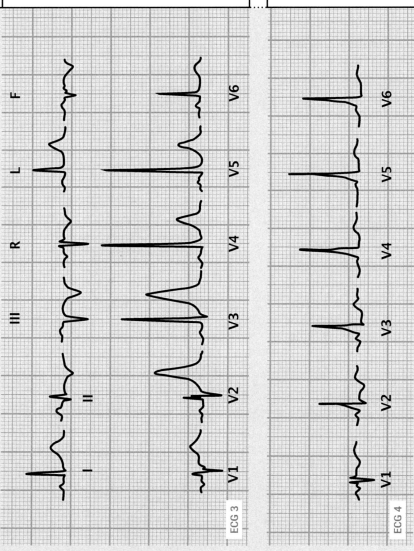

ECG 3

ECG 4

PR	1° AV block	
	WPW syndrome	
	LGL syndrome	
QRS duration	Complete RBBB	
	Complete LBBB	
	Dilated right ventricle	
	Dilated left ventricle	
Rotation	Normal transition zone	
	Clockwise rotation	
	Counterclockwise rotation	
Hyper-trophy	Right ventricular hypertrophy	
	Left ventricular hypertrophy	
Infarction	Anteroseptal region	
	Anterior wall	
	Anterolateral region	
	Lateral region	
	Posterolateral region	
	Posterior wall	
	Inferior wall	

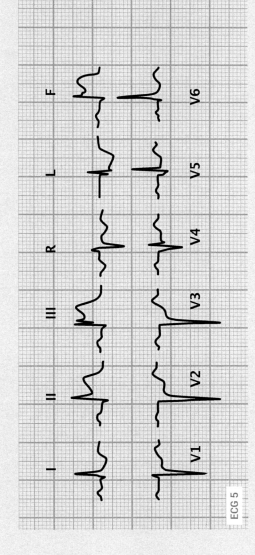

ECG 5

Level 10

Acute coronary syndromes—mastering the ST segment

"Wisdom...comes not from age,
but from education and learning."
—Anton Chekhov

Acute coronary syndromes—mastering the ST segment

In this chapter you'll learn about the acute coronary syndromes and how they affect the ST segment.

The acute coronary syndromes

In the previous chapters we discussed what happens to the QRS complex in the setting of myocardial infarction. You learned that the QRS complex "drowns in negativity" when myocardial infarction occurs, which means that R-wave amplitudes decrease and Q waves emerge.

These QRS changes are signs of myocardial necrosis and/or scarring. Scars are usually irreversible, so these changes to the QRS complex are also **irreversible**.

However, myocardial infarction not only affects the QRS complex but also the ST segment, and these changes are usually **transient**.

Acute myocardial infarction is part of the so-called **acute coronary syndromes** (ACS). Acute coronary syndromes result from coronary arteries that are (partly) occluded either by a thrombus or ruptured plaque.

If you want to become a true master of the ST segment, you'll need a thorough understanding of the different acute coronary syndromes. So here they are.

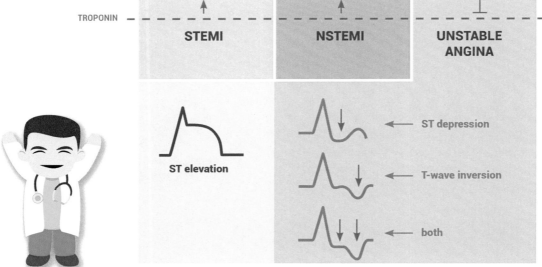

STEMI = ST elevation myocardial infarction
NSTEMI = non-STEMI

A few things to remember:

1. Both **STEMIs** and **NSTEMIs** are characterized by an **elevation of troponin** in the blood. Troponin is elevated because myocardial cells are dying off.

2. As the name implies, **STEMI** comes with an **elevation of the ST segment** (duh!), which discriminates it from NSTEMI and unstable angina.

3. In **NSTEMI and unstable angina**, changes to the ST segment can be subtle; there can be **ST depression, T-wave inversion**, or both.

4. ST changes are very similar in unstable angina and NSTEMI. However, in **unstable angina, troponin** (and other cardiac enzymes) are **NOT elevated**.

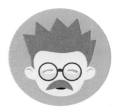

The terms "STEMI," "acute myocardial infarction," and "ACS with ST elevation" are sometimes used interchangeably. However, ACS doesn't necessarily lead to myocardial infarction (i.e., necrosis). Therefore, you should think of ST elevation as a sign of acute ischemia rather than infarction, although in general it is its first step.

The figure below shows the different pathways and different stages of acute coronary syndromes.

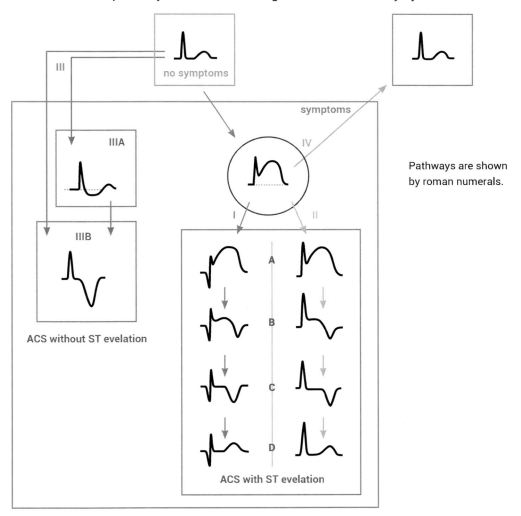

Pathways are shown by roman numerals.

Pathways I and II—ACS with ST elevation

We start off with the normal heart, shown in yellow.

As symptoms develop, **ST-segment elevation appears** (ischemia). Now three pathways are possible (I, II, and IV). Let's first take a look at ST elevations with Q waves (pathway I in the previous illustration).

A few hours after the beginning of myocardial ischemia, pathologic **Q waves appear** as a sign of necrosis (IA in the illustration).

As mentioned above, ST elevation is a transient phenomenon. The process from ST elevation to its resolution is called **ST-segment resolution**. It starts with the ST segment going down and the T wave becoming negative (IB).

In the subacute phase of myocardial infarction (IC), the **ST segment has returned to the isoelectric line**, and **the T wave has become negative**. In some patients, this pattern persists forever.

In the chronic phase of myocardial infarction (ID), the T wave becomes positive again. There is no residual sign of infarction in the ST segment or T wave. The myocardial scar is only visible as a Q wave or QS complex.

Time until complete ST-segment resolution is variable. It strongly depends on time to revascularization. Usually, the ST segment starts to go down immediately after complete revascularization. In other cases ST elevation disappears only after several days. Persistence of ST-segment elevations for weeks after myocardial infarction is alarming as it is often caused by a left ventricular aneurysm.

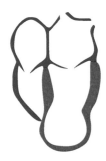

myocardial aneurysm

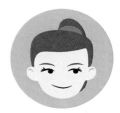

The time-dependent pattern of changes seen in the ST segment and T wave can also be observed in non−Q-wave infarction (and in patients with perimyocarditis)—this is pathway II in the illustration.

Pathway III—ACS without ST elevation

In NSTEMI and unstable angina, symptoms are associated with ST depression (IIIA in the illustration) or T-wave inversion (IIIB). To differentiate between NSTEMI and unstable angina, you'll have to look at whether cardiac enzymes are elevated.

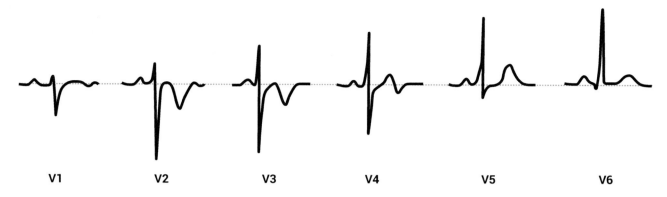

V1 **V2** **V3** **V4** **V5** **V6**

NSTEMI in the territory of the left anterior descending artery (LAD). Leads V2, V3, and V4 are affected. Could also be diagnosed as unstable angina if troponin stays within normal limits.

Pathway IV—Prinzmetal angina: a special case

There is a form of myocardial ischemia that's commonly associated with ST elevation. This disease is called **variant angina** or **Prinzmetal angina**. Chest pain is typically of short duration (15 to 20 minutes) and appears at rest or even during sleep. Unlike other forms of angina, ST elevation returns to baseline immediately after symptoms disappear. Coronary occlusion is thought to be caused by coronary spasm in these cases.

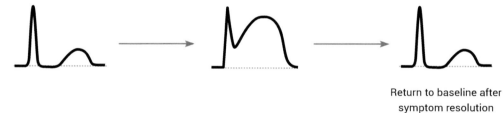

Return to baseline after symptom resolution

Perimyocarditis

In perimyocarditis, the ST segment is usually also elevated and shows the stages we have seen in IIA through IID. Perimyocarditis is a diffuse disease, and unlike infarction, it's not limited to the perfusion territory of one coronary artery. So it can be seen in most limb leads and many of the precordial leads.

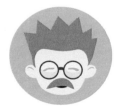

Whenever you see ST elevations in areas that are not supplied by one single artery, you should think of perimyocarditis.

Typically, the ST elevation is not convex, as in myocardial infarction, but rather concave (as seen in the following figure). Furthermore, the ST segment usually originates from the ascending part of the QRS complex in perimyocarditis, whereas in STEMI it usually originates from the descending part of the QRS.

Perimyocarditis

STEMI

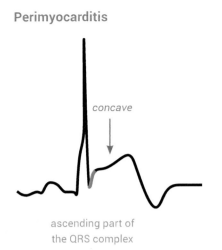

concave

convex

ascending part of
the QRS complex

descending part of the QRS complex

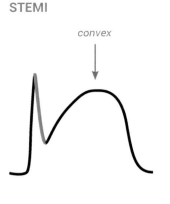

In perimyocarditis you can also see the time-dependent changes in ACS with ST elevation, ST resolution, T-wave inversion, etc.

Vagotonia

And finally, there's one more form of ST-segment elevation that's rather innocent compared with the previous ones. This type of ST elevation can be seen in the setting of vagotonia (i.e., an increase in vagal tone). The elevation is up to 0.2 mV in amplitude, and it's usually accompanied by a tall and peaked T wave, as well as a low heart rate of <60 beats per minute.

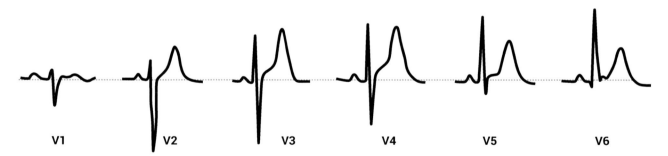

V1　　**V2**　　**V3**　　**V4**　　**V5**　　**V6**

Case of vagotonia with ST elevation and a tall, peaked T wave.

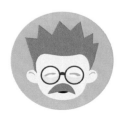

With this knowledge in mind, we can now add the evaluation of the ST segment to the steps of our cookbook. Note that the ST segment should always be evaluated in combination with the QRS complex.

Question	Answer	Diagnosis
1. Rhythm	[coming later]	[coming later]
2. Heart rate	[coming later]	[coming later]
3. P waves	[coming later]	[coming later]
4. PR interval	a) >0.2 s (if PR interval constant for all beats and each P wave is followed by a QRS complex)	I° AV block
	b) <0.12 s and QRS complex normal	LGL syndrome
	c) <0.12 s and visible delta wave	WPW syndrome
5. QRS axis	Determine the axis according to leads I, II, and aVF	normal axis left axis deviation right axis deviation north–west axis
6. QRS duration	a) ≥0.12 s (always think of WPW syndrome as a differential)	complete bundle branch block
	b) >0.1 s and <0.12 s with typical bundle branch block appearance (notching)	incomplete bundle branch block
7. Rotation	Rotation is defined according to the heart's transition zone. Normally the transition zone is located at V4, which means that right ventricular myocardium is located at V1–V3 and left ventricular myocardium is at V5–V6.	transition zone at V5–V6: clockwise rotation transition zone at V1–V3: counterclockwise rotation NOTE: don't evaluate rotation in the setting of myocardial infarction, WPW syndrome, or bundle branch block
8. QRS amplitude	a) QRS amplitude <0.5 mV in all standard leads	low voltage
	b) Positive criteria for left ventricular hypertrophy	left ventricular hypertrophy
	c) Positive criteria for right ventricular hypertrophy	right ventricular hypertrophy
9. QRS infarction signs	abnormal Q waves, QS waves, missing R-wave progression	myocardial infarction; localization according to affected leads

10. ST-T segment

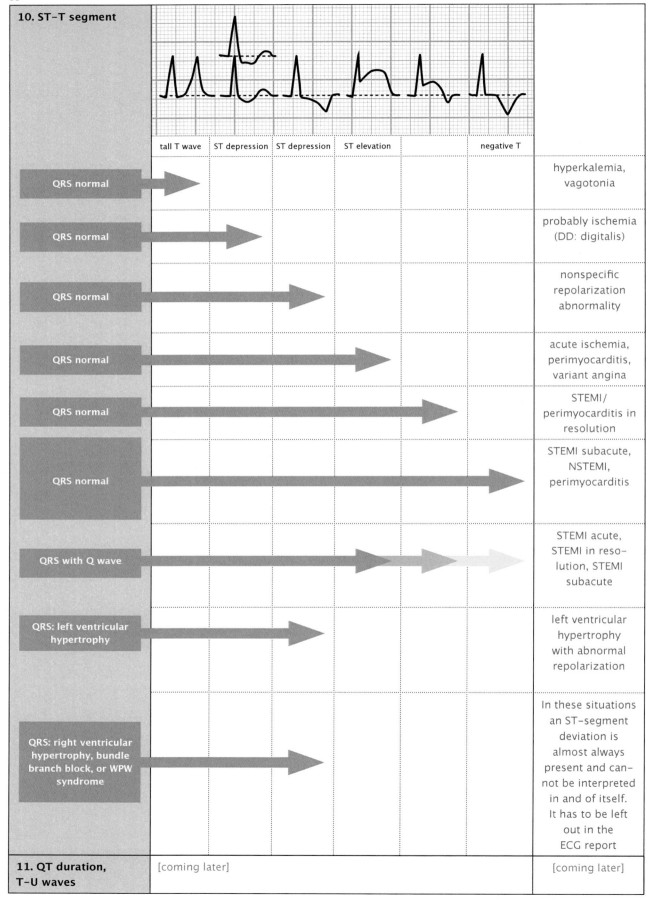

	tall T wave	ST depression	ST depression	ST elevation		negative T	
QRS normal	→						hyperkalemia, vagotonia
QRS normal		→					probably ischemia (DD: digitalis)
QRS normal			→				nonspecific repolarization abnormality
QRS normal				→			acute ischemia, perimyocarditis, variant angina
QRS normal					→		STEMI/ perimyocarditis in resolution
QRS normal						→	STEMI subacute, NSTEMI, perimyocarditis
QRS with Q wave				→	→	→	STEMI acute, STEMI in reso-lution, STEMI subacute
QRS: left ventricular hypertrophy			→				left ventricular hypertrophy with abnormal repolarization
QRS: right ventricular hypertrophy, bundle branch block, or WPW syndrome			→				In these situations an ST–segment deviation is almost always present and can-not be interpreted in and of itself. It has to be left out in the ECG report

11. QT duration, T–U waves | [coming later] | | | | | | [coming later] |

Level 10

QUIZ SECTION

For the following exercises, use our cookbook including the evaluation of the ST segment.

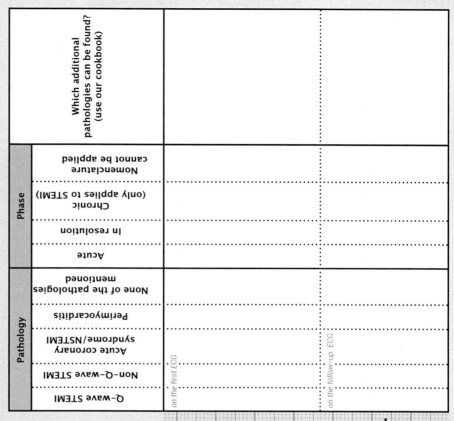

	Pathology					Phase				Which additional pathologies can be found? (use our cookbook)
	Q-wave STEMI	Non-Q-wave STEMI	Acute coronary syndrome/NSTEMI	Perimyocarditis	None of the pathologies mentioned	Acute	In resolution	Chronic (only applies to STEMI)	Nomenclature cannot be applied	
on the first ECG										
on the follow-up ECG										

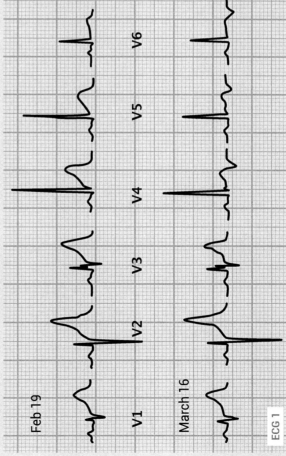

Feb 19

V1 V2 V3 V4 V5 V6

March 16

ECG 1

Pathology					Phase				Which additional pathologies can be found? (use our cookbook)
Q-wave STEMI	Non-Q-wave STEMI	Acute coronary syndrome/NSTEMI	Perimyocarditis	None of the pathologies mentioned	Acute	In resolution	Chronic (only applies to STEMI)	Nomenclature cannot be applied	

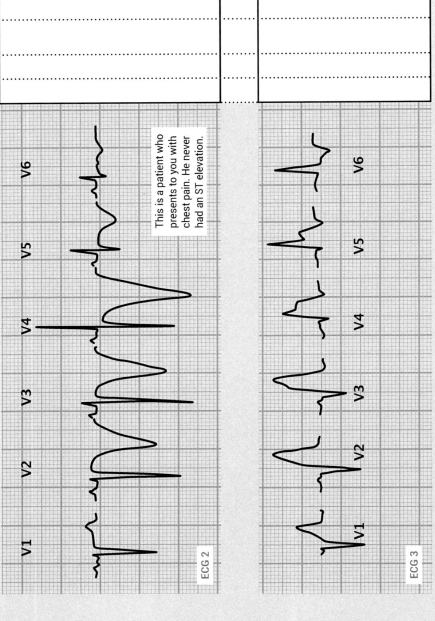

This is a patient who presents to you with chest pain. He never had an ST elevation.

ECG 2

ECG 3

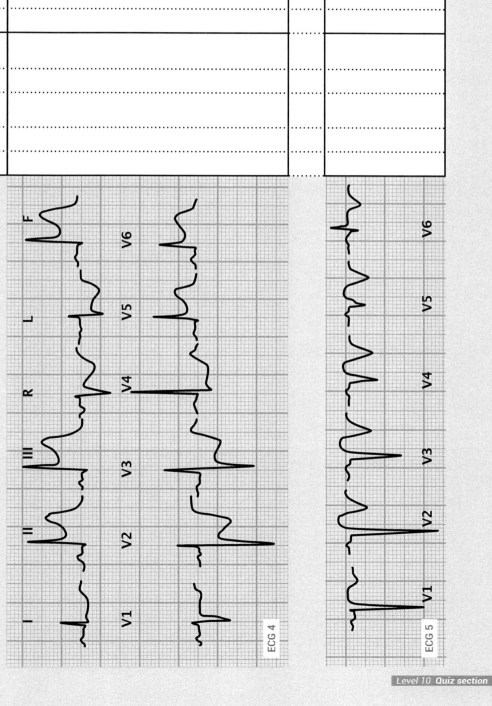

Pathology					Phase				Which additional pathologies can be found? (use our cookbook)
Q-wave STEMI	Non-Q-wave STEMI	Acute coronary syndrome/NSTEMI	Perimyocarditis	None of the pathologies mentioned	Acute	In resolution	Chronic (only applies to STEMI)	Nomenclature cannot be applied	

ECG 4

ECG 5

	Pathology					Phase				Which additional pathologies can be found? (use our cookbook)
	Q-wave STEMI	Non-Q-wave STEMI	Acute coronary syndrome/NSTEMI	Perimyocarditis	None of the pathologies mentioned	Acute	In resolution	Chronic (only applies to STEMI)	Nomenclature cannot be applied	
ECG 6										
ECG 7										

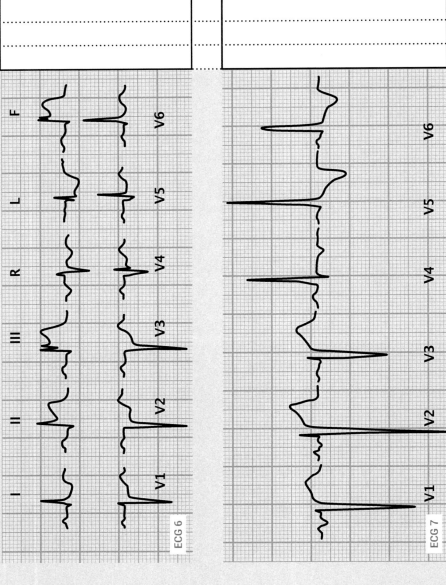

ECG 6

ECG 7

Pathology					Phase				Which additional pathologies can be found? (use our cookbook)
Q-wave STEMI	Non-Q-wave STEMI	Acute coronary syndrome/NSTEMI	Perimyocarditis	None of the pathologies mentioned	Acute	In resolution	Chronic (only applies to STEMI)	Nomenclature cannot be applied	

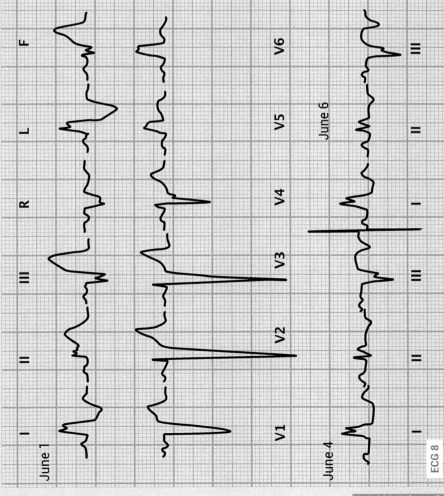

ECG 8

The ECG trio—cardiac axis, atrial hypertrophy, and low voltage

"Any fool can know. The point is to understand."
—Albert Einstein

The ECG trio—cardiac axis, atrial hypertrophy, and low voltage

In this chapter, you will learn an easy and fast method for how to determine the cardiac axis. The good news is, it's much easier than everyone tells you.

The shocking truth about the cardiac axis

If you're like most ECG students, you find the evaluation of the cardiac axis utterly confusing, and you are not sure why you have to learn it at all. Quite frankly, you are absolutely right.

When you compare the amount of time most folks spend studying the axis and the actual value it adds to their reports, you'll notice that the return on their time is humble. The good news is that there are only a couple of things that are really important about the axis. In this section, we'll teach you what they are.

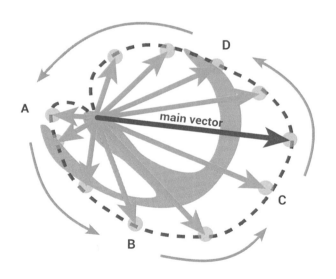

With the complicated geometry of the ventricles, you can imagine that at each point in time there are vectors of different amplitudes pointing in different directions inside the heart. From all these momentary vectors, an average vector can be constructed for each point in time.

We know that ventricular depolarization takes about 80 to 100 ms (<0.1 s). In this image we have marked a few of these instantaneous average vectors: A: vector at 5 ms; B: vector at 30 ms; C: vector at 60 ms; D: vector at 80 ms. The dashed line connecting the tips of these vectors represents the vector loop.

The strongest (i.e., longest) of these average vectors is called the **main vector**; it is the one that determines the electrical axis of the heart in the frontal plane. In other words, the cardiac axis represents the direction of the main electrical vector in the frontal plane.

The most precise way to determine the axis in the frontal plane would be to exactly calculate the direction of the main vector. However, that's too time consuming and not worth the effort because there are only a few situations in which knowledge of the axis really makes a difference. You'll learn what they are a little later.

What we should be able to do is to find the most important abnormalities of the electrical axis. Next we outline a simple trick for doing so.

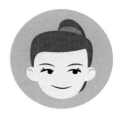

*Remember that a lead records a **positive wave** when the **vector points into the direction of that lead**. When the **vector points away from that lead**, the deflection will be mainly **negative**.*

First, we have to learn the location of the leads (I, II, III, aVR, aVL, and aVF) on the Cabrera circle (or Cabrera system). This system provides a convention for representing the limb leads in a logical sequence. The location of each lead can be seen in the image below.

The degrees of the circle start near lead I with 0. When we go clockwise, the degrees are +60°, +90°, etc., and when we go counterclockwise they are negative (-30°, etc.).

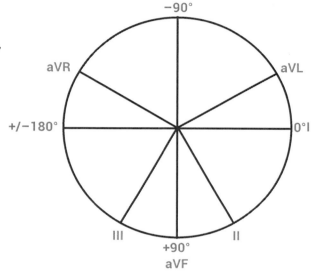

Let us now consider what this means for lead I:

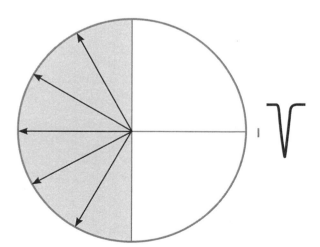

Deflection is **negative** when vectors point **away from** lead I

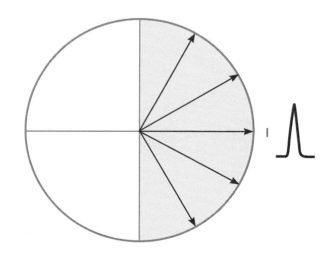

Deflection is **positive** when vectors point **in the direction** of lead I

Let's see what happens when leads I and II are mainly positive:

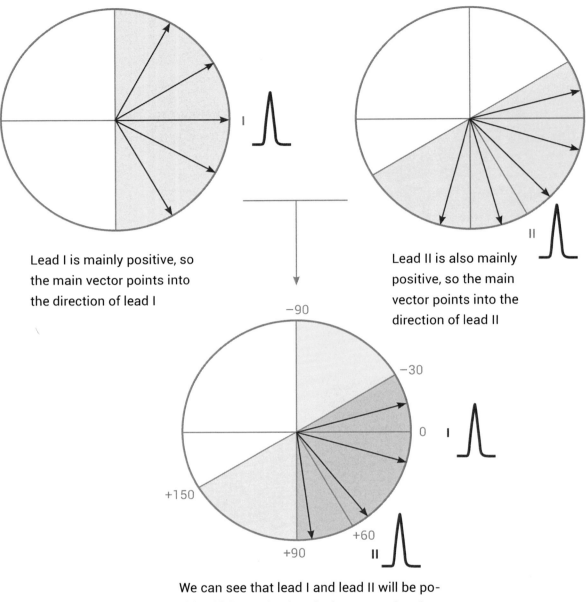

Lead I is mainly positive, so the main vector points into the direction of lead I

Lead II is also mainly positive, so the main vector points into the direction of lead II

We can see that lead I and lead II will be positive if the main electrical vector points into the intersection of the yellow and blue areas

The area between −30° and +90° is called a "normal axis"

So we know that if leads I and II are positive, the vector points at the area between −30° to +90°. Most electrical vectors in humans are located in that sector and that's why we call it a normal axis. The terminology varies in different medical schools and countries. We will use the terms mostly used in British and American textbooks.

Now let's see what happens when lead I is positive and lead II is negative:

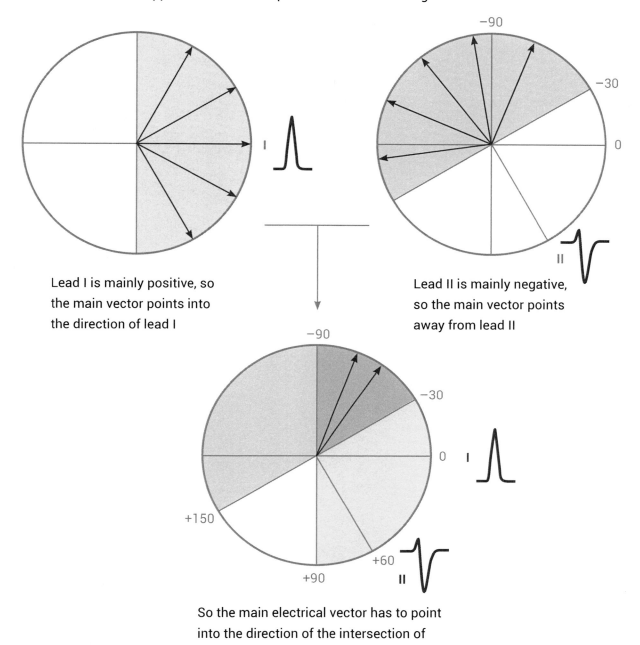

Lead I is mainly positive, so
the main vector points into
the direction of lead I

Lead II is mainly negative,
so the main vector points
away from lead II

So the main electrical vector has to point
into the direction of the intersection of
the yellow and gray areas

The area between −30° and −90° is called "left axis deviation"

If lead I is negative, you should look at lead aVF instead of lead II to determine the axis.

Now let's see what happens when lead I is negative and aVF is positive:

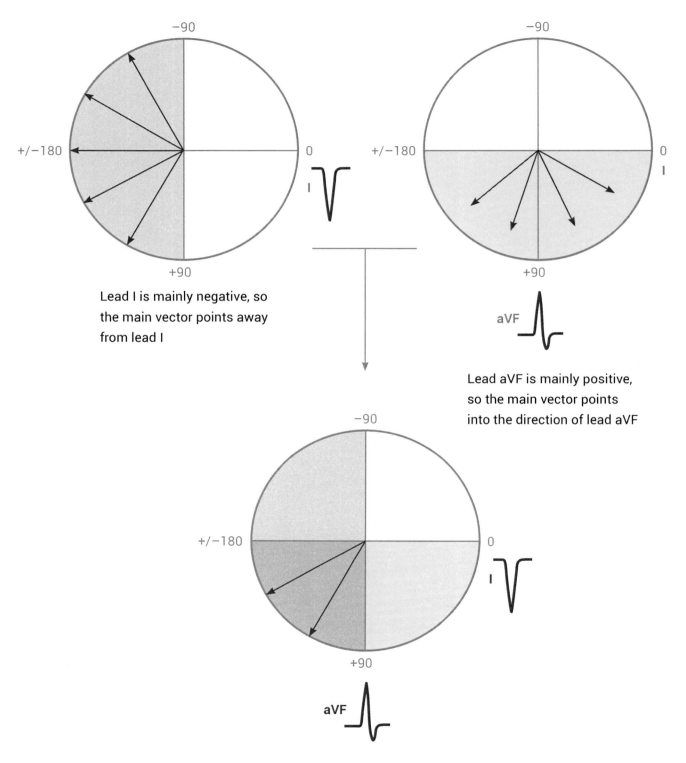

Lead I is mainly negative, so the main vector points away from lead I

Lead aVF is mainly positive, so the main vector points into the direction of lead aVF

The main vector has to point at the intersection of the gray and blue areas

The area between +90° and +/−180° is called "right axis deviation"

And what's the matter when both leads I and aVF are negative?

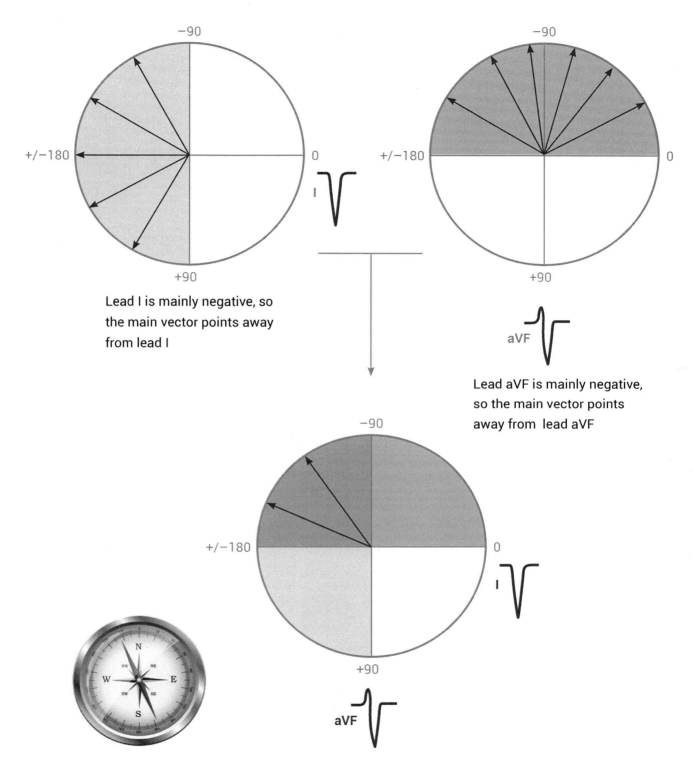

Lead I is mainly negative, so the main vector points away from lead I

Lead aVF is mainly negative, so the main vector points away from lead aVF

The main vector has to point at the intersection of the grey and blue areas

The area between −90° and +/−180° is called a "northwest axis"

You should only care about left axis deviation and right axis deviation for now. Why? Because when the axis is normal, that won't really help you in refining your diagnosis. A northwest axis is extremely rare—you won't encounter it much as a novice. But you will encounter left axis deviation and right axis deviation, and they will help you in your diagnosis.

So here's an overview:

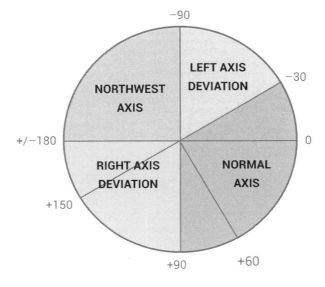

So how can you determine the cardiac axis really easily? Here's how...

All you have to do to determine the cardiac axis is to hold the ECG printout in your hands. Your left thumb should be next to lead I. **If lead I is positive, lead II should be next to your right thumb. If lead I is mainly negative, lead aVF should be next to your right thumb:**

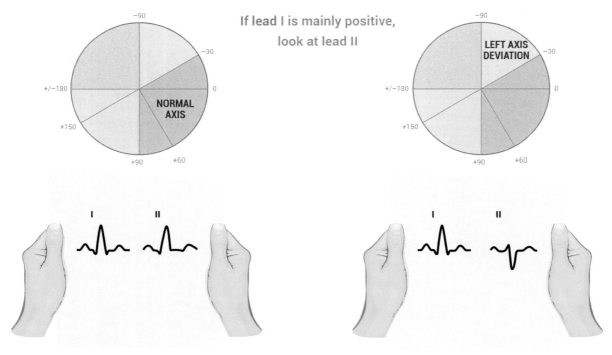

If both leads are mainly positive,
it's a **normal axis**

If the left lead is mainly positive and the right
lead is mainly negative, it's a **left axis deviation**

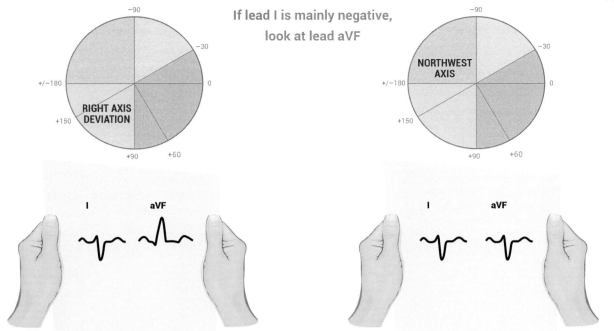

If lead I is mainly negative, look at lead aVF

If the right lead is mainly positive and the left lead is mainly negative, it's **right axis deviation**

If both leads are mainly negative, it's a **northwest axis**

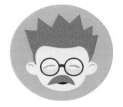

You'll get plenty of opportunities to assess the axis in the exercises!

Now let's turn to the clinical situations in which knowledge of the cardiac axis makes a difference.

Situation #1

For ventricular depolarization, impulses are conducted down into the ventricles through the so-called bundle branches. There's a right bundle branch (RBB) and a left bundle branch (LBB). The left bundle branch is subdivided into a left anterior fascicle (LAF) and a left posterior fascicle (LPF) as shown in the image:

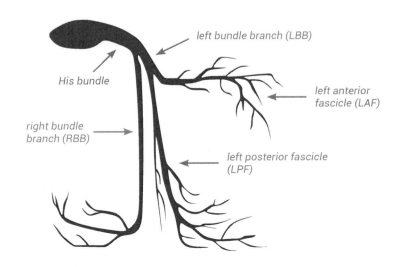

We have already learned that the QRS complex broadens when either the right or the left bundle branch is blocked. Sometimes what happens in right bundle branch block is that one of the left fascicles is also blocked. That's called a bifascicular block. It's a pretty dangerous situation because there's only one fascicle that's left for the impulse to reach the ventricles. If this last fascicle gets blocked as well, the patient ends up in complete heart block, a potentially life-threatening situation.

How can you tell whether bifascicular block is present? Well, if you have a typical picture of a right bundle branch block in the precordial leads and you also have left axis deviation, the patient has bifascicular block involving the left anterior fascicle (also called "right bundle branch block with left anterior hemiblock"):

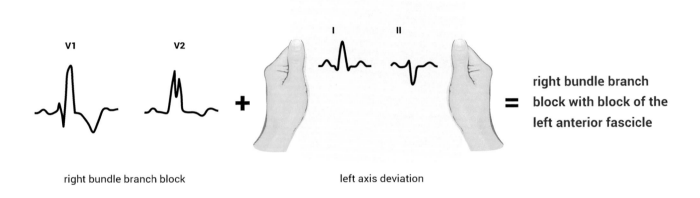

right bundle branch block   left axis deviation   right bundle branch block with block of the left anterior fascicle

The abbreviation for the left anterior fascicle is LAF. So there's a straightforward mnemonic for this situation:

Left axis deviation = LAF(T) block

When the patient has right bundle branch block plus right axis deviation, she probably also has bifascicular block with involvement of the left posterior fascicle:

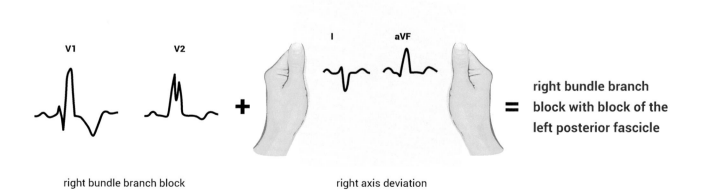

right bundle branch block   right axis deviation   right bundle branch block with block of the left posterior fascicle

Situation #2

Whenever you suspect right ventricular hypertrophy from looking at the precordial leads, it often helps to look for the presence of right axis deviation, which would reinforce your suspicion. So whenever the RSS criteria are positive (e.g., you have a patient with a tall R in V1 and a deep S in V5) and this patient also has right axis deviation, then you can be almost certain that something's wrong with the right heart:

signs of right ventricular hypertrophy in precordial leads **+** **right axis deviation** ⟶ **increases likelihood of right ventricular hypertrophy**

Situation #3

When there are signs of left ventricular hypertrophy in the ECG and the patient also has right axis deviation, you should think of biventricular hypertrophy. As the name implies, this is a situation in which both the left and the right ventricles are hypertrophic.

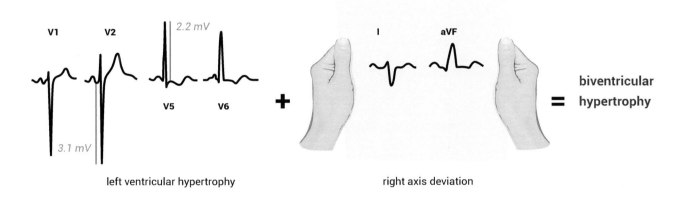

left ventricular hypertrophy + right axis deviation = biventricular hypertrophy

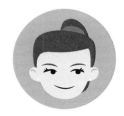

Great! Now you know when knowledge of the cardiac axis really makes a difference. You should now integrate the evaluation of cardiac axis into the steps of the cookbook. Congrats, you've almost made it through the training!

Atrial hypertrophy

Hypertrophy of the atria can be evaluated by looking at the P waves in the standard leads.

Left atrial hypertrophy

The P wave has two peaks, and usually the second peak is taller than the first one. P-wave duration is greater than 0.1 seconds. These changes are most pronounced in leads I and II. This type of P wave is called **P mitrale**:

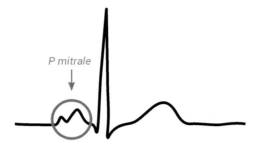

P mitrale can also be nicely depicted in lead V1, where we would typically see a biphasic (i.e., positive–negative) P wave. The negative part of the P wave corresponds to the enlarged left atrium. If the negative part is longer than 1 small box (or >0.04 s), then P mitrale is present:

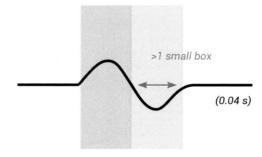

Right atrial hypertrophy

This is best seen in leads II, III, and aVF. The P wave is peaked and exceeds 0.25 mV in amplitude. These peaked P waves are called **P pulmonale.**

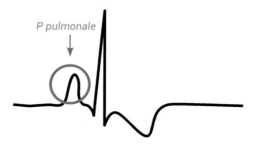

Here are the criteria again:

	V1	II	criteria
Normal			
right atrial enlargement P pulmonale			P > 2.5 mm in II
left atrial enlargement P mitrale			negative P in V1 >0.04 s and/or P-wave duration >0.12 s in most cases

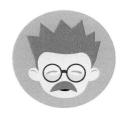

With this knowledge in mind, you should now add the evaluation of P waves to your cookbook approach!

Low voltage

Low voltage refers to a situation in which none of the QRS complexes in the standard leads (i.e., leads I, II, and III) is higher than 0.5 mV. Possible reasons for this finding are peripheral edema, pulmonary emphysema, large pericardial effusion, or severe myocardial damage, among others. The ECG cannot provide you with a definitive diagnosis; it can just give you a hint that further workups are necessary.

Question	Answer	Diagnosis
1. Rhythm	[coming later]	[coming later]
2. Heart rate	[coming later]	[coming later]
3. P waves	a) Large P-wave amplitude (>2.5 mm in II, III, or aVF)	right atrial enlargement
	b) Prolonged negative part of P wave in V1 (1 mm) and P wave with 2 peaks in II, P-wave duration >0.12 s	left atrial enlargement
4. PR interval	a) >0.2 s (if PR interval constant for all beats and each P wave is followed by a QRS complex)	I° AV block
	b) <0.12 s and QRS complex normal	LGL syndrome
	c) <0.12 s and visible delta wave	WPW syndrome
5. QRS axis	Determine the axis according to leads I, II, and aVF	normal axis left axis deviation right axis deviation north-west axis
6. QRS duration	a) ≥0.12 s (always think of WPW syndrome as a differential)	complete bundle branch block
	b) >0.1 s and <0.12 s with typical bundle branch block appearance (notching)	incomplete bundle branch block
7. Rotation	Rotation is defined according to the heart's transition zone. Normally the transition zone is located at V4, which means that right ventricular myocardium is located at V1–V3 and left ventricular myocardium is at V5–V6.	transition zone at V5–V6: clockwise rotation transition zone at V1–V3: counterclockwise rotation NOTE: don't evaluate rotation in the setting of myocardial infarction, WPW syndrome, or bundle branch block
8. QRS amplitude	a) QRS amplitude <0.5 mV in all standard leads	low voltage
	b) Positive criteria for left ventricular hypertrophy	left ventricular hypertrophy
	c) Positive criteria for right ventricular hypertrophy	right ventricular hypertrophy
9. QRS infarction signs	abnormal Q waves, QS waves, missing R-wave progression	myocardial infarction; localization according to affected leads

10. ST–T segment							

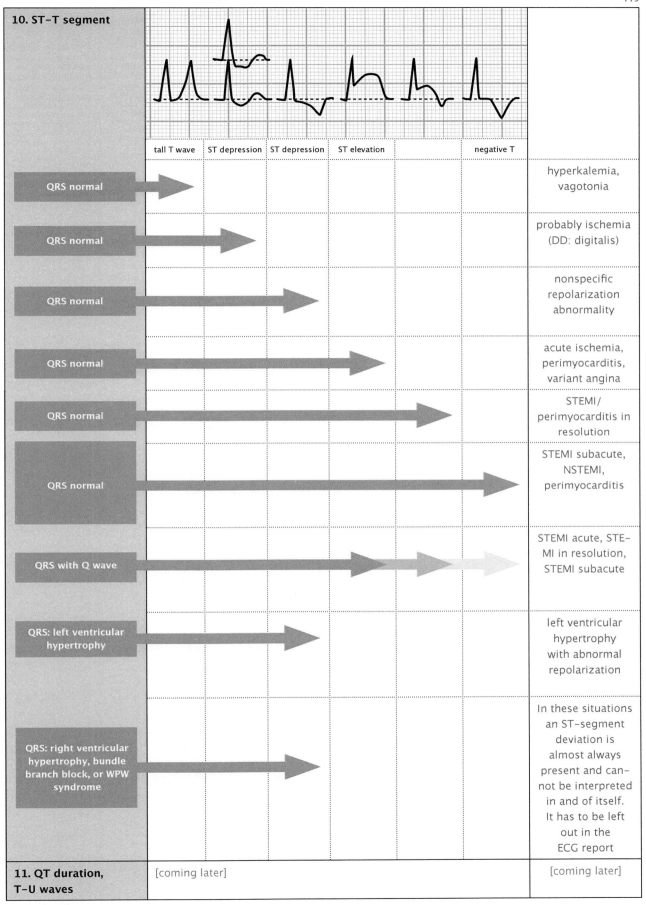

	tall T wave	ST depression	ST depression	ST elevation		negative T	
QRS normal	→						hyperkalemia, vagotonia
QRS normal		→					probably ischemia (DD: digitalis)
QRS normal			→				nonspecific repolarization abnormality
QRS normal				→			acute ischemia, perimyocarditis, variant angina
QRS normal					→		STEMI/ perimyocarditis in resolution
QRS normal						→	STEMI subacute, NSTEMI, perimyocarditis
QRS with Q wave				→	→	→	STEMI acute, STE-MI in resolution, STEMI subacute
QRS: left ventricular hypertrophy			→				left ventricular hypertrophy with abnormal repolarization
QRS: right ventricular hypertrophy, bundle branch block, or WPW syndrome			→				In these situations an ST–segment deviation is almost always present and can-not be interpreted in and of itself. It has to be left out in the ECG report
11. QT duration, T–U waves	[coming later]						[coming later]

Level 11

QUIZ SECTION

And now it's time for some exercises...

	Electrical axis	Which additional changes can be found? (use our cookbook!)
Normal axis		
Left axis deviation		
Right axis deviation		
northwest axis / extreme axis deviation		

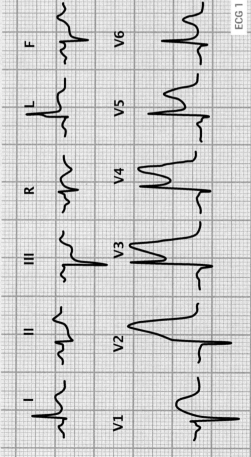

ECG 1

Electrical axis		Which additional changes can be found? (use our cookbook!)
Normal axis		
Left axis deviation		
Right axis deviation		
northwest axis/ extreme axis deviation		

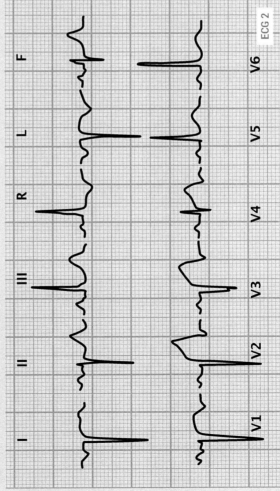

ECG 2

Electrical axis				Which additional changes can be found? (use our cookbook!)
Normal axis	Left axis deviation	Right axis deviation	northwest axis / extreme axis deviation	

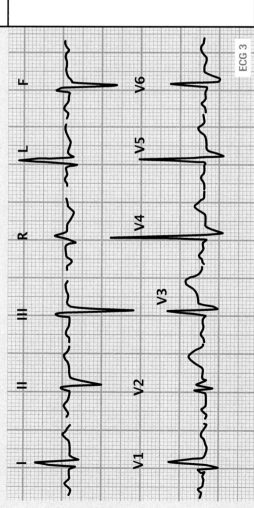

ECG 3

Electrical axis				Which additional changes can be found? (use our cookbook!)
Normal axis	Left axis deviation	Right axis deviation	northwest axis / extreme axis deviation	

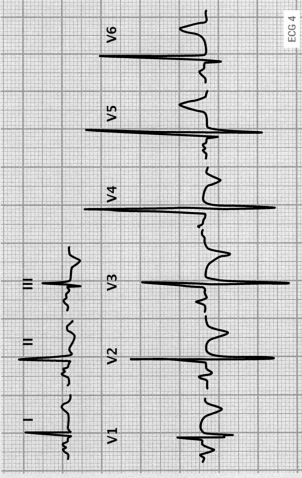

ECG 4

Which additional changes can be found? (use our cookbook!)	Electrical axis			
	Normal axis	Left axis deviation	Right axis deviation	northwest axis / extreme axis deviation

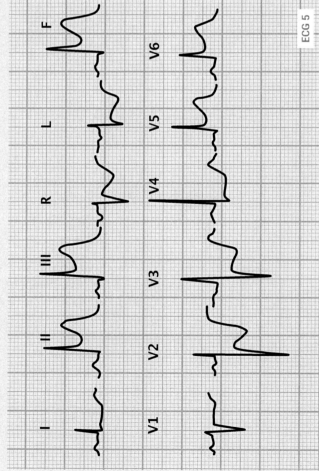

ECG 5

Electrical axis				Which additional changes can be found? (use our cookbook!)
Normal axis	Left axis deviation	Right axis deviation	northwest axis/ extreme axis deviation	

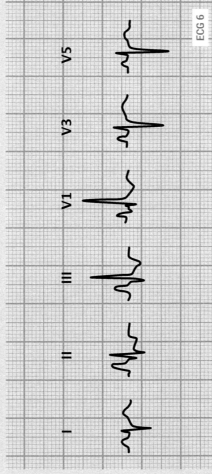

ECG 6

Level 12

A short story about electrolytes and heart rate

"I am learning all the time. The tombstone will be my diploma."
—Eartha Kitt

A short story about electrolytes and heart rate

The ECG can help you detect various kinds of electrolyte disturbances. Some of them are potentially life threatening.

Hyperkalemia and hypokalemia

Hyperkalemia (as seen in renal failure) is characterized by a **tall and "tented" T wave** (A in the illustration below). Sometimes the ECG can lead to a diagnosis of chronic renal failure even in patients who don't exhibit any symptoms yet. In more severe cases (B in the illustration), the **P wave gets lost** and the **QRS complex gets broader**.

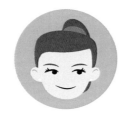

Remember that in vagotonia we can also see tall T waves. But these T waves are not as tall and sharp as the ones seen in hyperkalemia. Measurement of potassium levels will give you the answer.

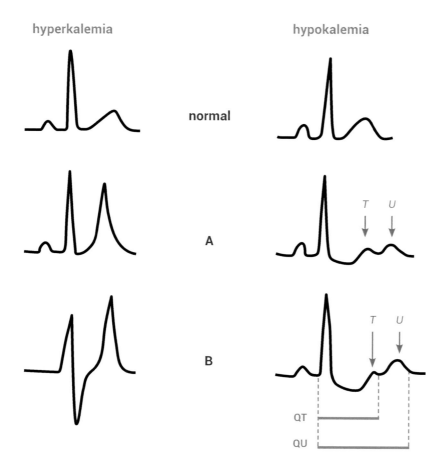

ECG changes seen in hypokalemia are a sign of cellular potassium loss. They are seen even before blood levels start to drop. That's why ECG changes associated with hypokalemia correlate less well with potassium levels than changes associated with hyperkalemia.

The typical ECG changes seen in **hypokalemia** are **flattening of the T wave, appearance of a U wave**, and **ST depression**. A U wave is a second positive deflection that comes after the T wave. Note that hypokalemia does not lead to a prolongation of the QT interval. The QT interval starts at the beginning of the QRS complex and ends at the end of the T wave.

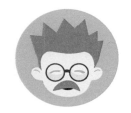

Don't confuse the QU interval with the QT interval!

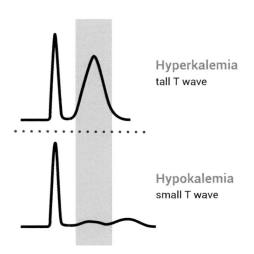

Hyperkalemia
tall T wave

Hypokalemia
small T wave

So remember:

- Hyperkalemia = tall T
- Hypokalemia = small T

Hypocalcemia and hypercalcemia

In hypercalcemia, the QT interval can be shortened, whereas in hypocalcemia, the QT interval can be prolonged.

And how will you know whether a patient's QT interval is normal or not? Well, the normal QT time varies with heart rate. **When heart rate is fast, the QT time shortens. When heart rate is slow, QT time becomes longer.** So there's no single normal value.

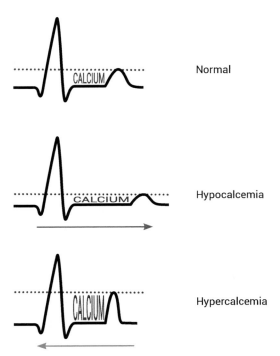

Normal

Hypocalcemia

Hypercalcemia

So how can you know whether your patient's QT interval is normal or not? There are two approaches that you should know for now:

1. Most ECG machines will calculate the QTc time for you. That's the corrected QT interval normalized for a heart rate of 60 beats/min. The QTc is prolonged if it's >0.44 seconds in men and >0.46 seconds in women.

2. And the quick and dirty method goes like this:

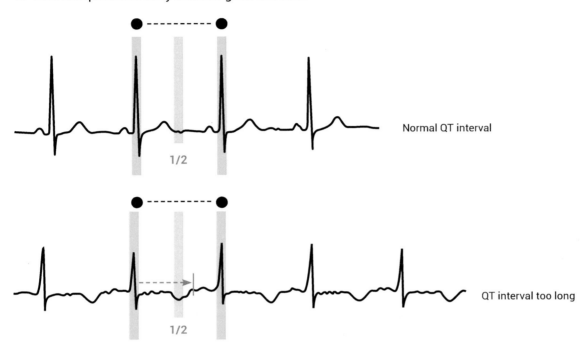

Normal QT interval

1/2

QT interval too long

1/2

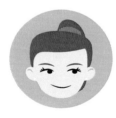

Take an RR interval and "cut" it in half. If the T wave ends in the first half of the RR interval (as in the top example), the QT interval is normal. If the T wave ends in the second half of the RR interval (as in the lower example), the QT time is prolonged. If the QT interval is prolonged, you should then calculate the QTc to verify your suspicion.

Heart rate quick tip

An easy way to assess heart rate is to divide 300 by the number of big boxes between two QRS complexes:

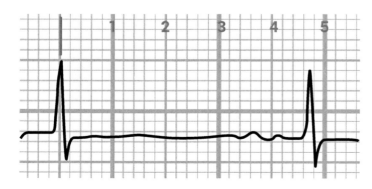

The distance from one QRS complex to the next is between 4 and 5 boxes in length. 300/4 would be 75 beats/min; 300/5 would be 60 beats/min. So the heart rate is between 75 and 60 (probably around 65 beats/min).

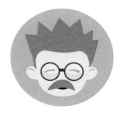

You should now add the evaluation of heart rate, T waves, U waves, and the QT interval into your cookbook approach!

Question	Answer	Diagnosis
1. Rhythm	[coming later]	[coming later]
2. Heart rate	Estimate heart rate: 300/number of large boxes between two QRS complexes	heart rate in beats per min
3. P waves	a) Large P-wave amplitude (>2.5 mm in II, III, or aVF)	right atrial enlargement
	b) Prolonged negative part of P wave in V1 (1 mm) and P wave with 2 peaks in II, P-wave duration >0.12 s	left atrial enlargement
4. PR interval	a) >0.2 s (if PR interval constant for all beats and each P wave is followed by a QRS complex)	I° AV block
	b) <0.12 s and QRS complex normal	LGL syndrome
	c) <0.12 s and visible delta wave	WPW syndrome
5. QRS axis	Determine the axis according to leads I, II, and aVF	normal axis left axis deviation right axis deviation northwest axis
6. QRS duration	a) ≥0.12 s (always think of WPW syndrome as a differential)	complete bundle branch block
	b) >0.1 s and <0.12 s with typical bundle branch block appearance (notching)	incomplete bundle branch block
7. Rotation	Rotation is defined according to the heart's transition zone. Normally the transition zone is located at V4, which means that right ventricular myocardium is located at V1–V3 and left ventricular myocardium is at V5–V6.	transition zone at V5–V6: clockwise rotation transition zone at V1–V3: counterclockwise rotation NOTE: don't evaluate rotation in the setting of myocardial infarction, WPW syndrome, or bundle branch block
8. QRS amplitude	a) QRS amplitude <0.5 mV in all standard leads	low voltage
	b) Positive criteria for left ventricular hypertrophy	left ventricular hypertrophy
	c) Positive criteria for right ventricular hypertrophy	right ventricular hypertrophy
9. QRS infarction signs	abnormal Q waves, QS waves, missing R-wave progression	myocardial infarction; localization according to affected leads

10. ST-T segment

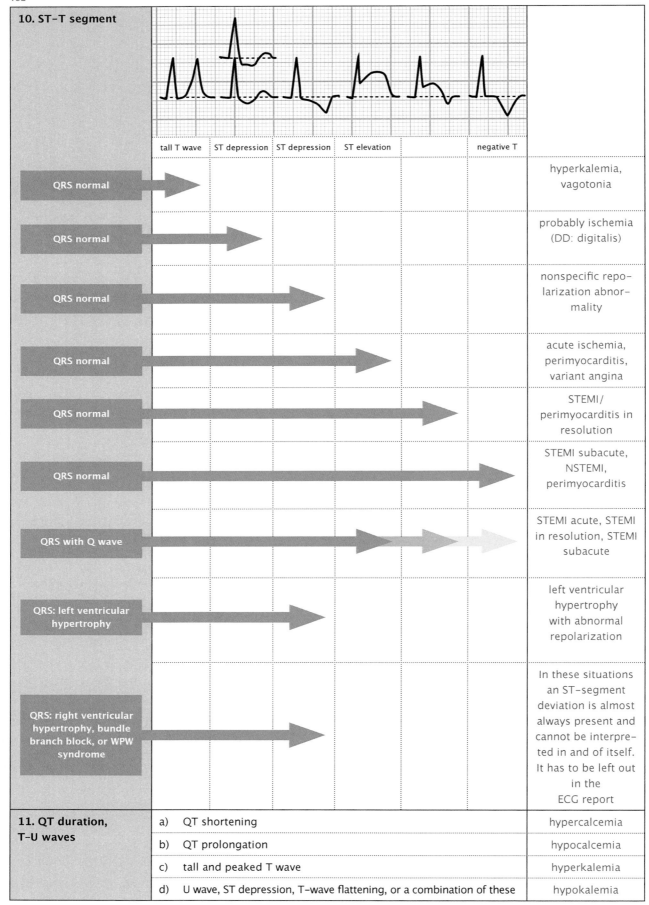

	tall T wave	ST depression	ST depression	ST elevation		negative T	
QRS normal	→						hyperkalemia, vagotonia
QRS normal		→					probably ischemia (DD: digitalis)
QRS normal			→				nonspecific repolarization abnormality
QRS normal				→			acute ischemia, perimyocarditis, variant angina
QRS normal					→		STEMI/ perimyocarditis in resolution
QRS normal						→	STEMI subacute, NSTEMI, perimyocarditis
QRS with Q wave				→	→	→	STEMI acute, STEMI in resolution, STEMI subacute
QRS: left ventricular hypertrophy			→				left ventricular hypertrophy with abnormal repolarization
QRS: right ventricular hypertrophy, bundle branch block, or WPW syndrome			→				In these situations an ST-segment deviation is almost always present and cannot be interpreted in and of itself. It has to be left out in the ECG report

11. QT duration, T-U waves

a)	QT shortening	hypercalcemia
b)	QT prolongation	hypocalcemia
c)	tall and peaked T wave	hyperkalemia
d)	U wave, ST depression, T-wave flattening, or a combination of these	hypokalemia

*Level 12 **A short story about electrolytes and heart rate***

Level 12

QUIZ SECTION

Please use the updated cookbook for the following exercises and go through all the steps that we have covered so far. (You can download the cookbook from www.medmastery.com, as described in the Introduction.) The numbers in the table below the ECGs correspond to the steps in the cookbook. If at one step during your evaluation you find that something is wrong (e.g., PR interval, QRS width, etc.), just tick off the respective number. You should estimate the heart rate and the axis for each ECG.

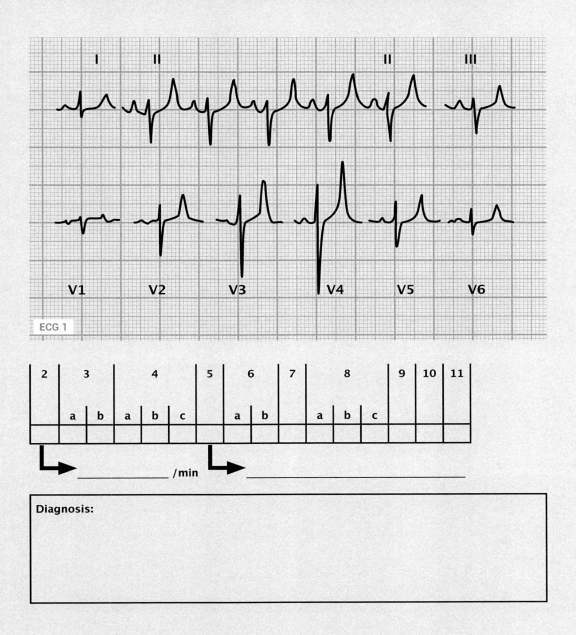

ECG 1

2	3		4		5	6		7	8			9	10	11
	a	b	a	b	c	a	b		a	b	c			

_____ /min   _____

Diagnosis:

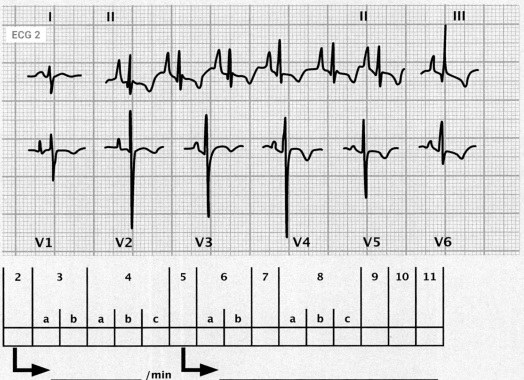

ECG 2

2	3		4			5	6	7	8			9	10	11
	a	b	a	b	c		a	b		a	b	c			

_____ /min   _____

Diagnosis:

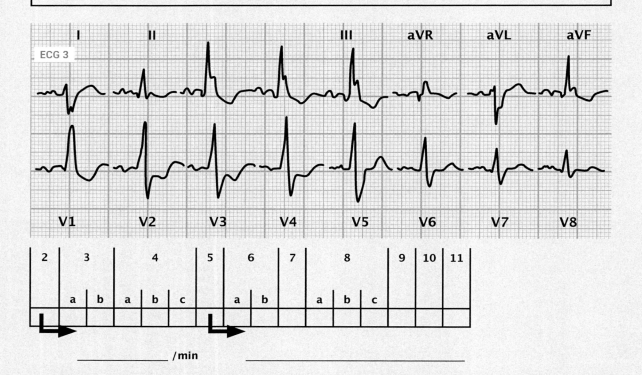

ECG 3

2	3		4			5	6	7	8			9	10	11
	a	b	a	b	c		a	b		a	b	c			

_____ /min   _____

Diagnosis:

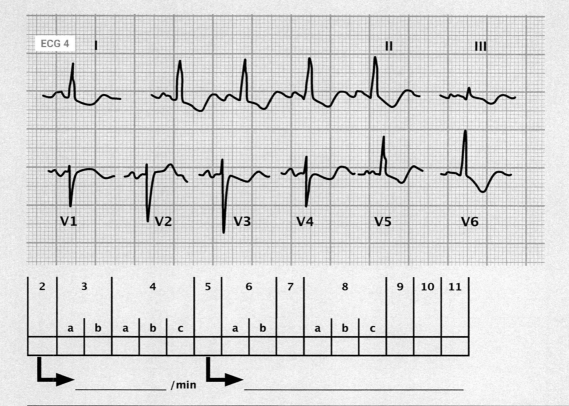

ECG 4

2	3		4			5	6		7	8			9	10	11
	a	b	a	b	c		a	b		a	b	c			

_____ /min   _____

Diagnosis:

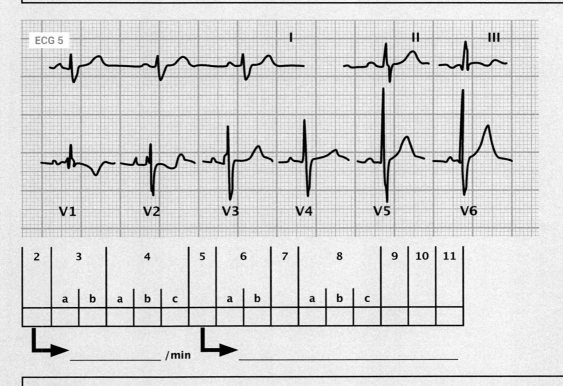

ECG 5

2	3		4			5	6		7	8			9	10	11
	a	b	a	b	c		a	b		a	b	c			

_____ /min   _____

Diagnosis:

ECG 6

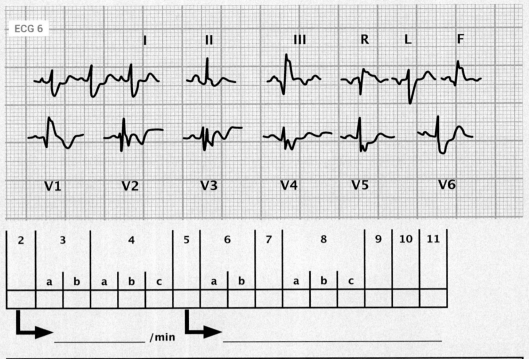

2	3		4			5	6		7	8			9	10	11
	a	b	a	b	c		a	b		a	b	c			

_____ /min

_____

Diagnosis:

ECG 7

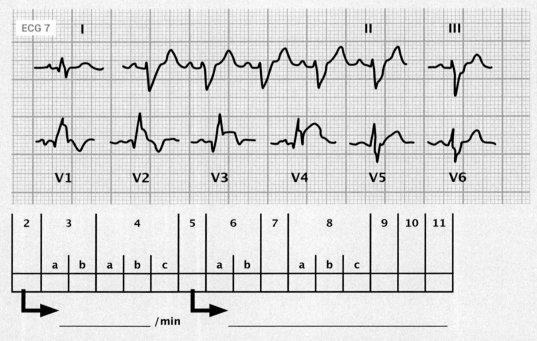

2	3		4			5	6		7	8			9	10	11
	a	b	a	b	c		a	b		a	b	c			

_____ /min

_____

Diagnosis:

ECG 8

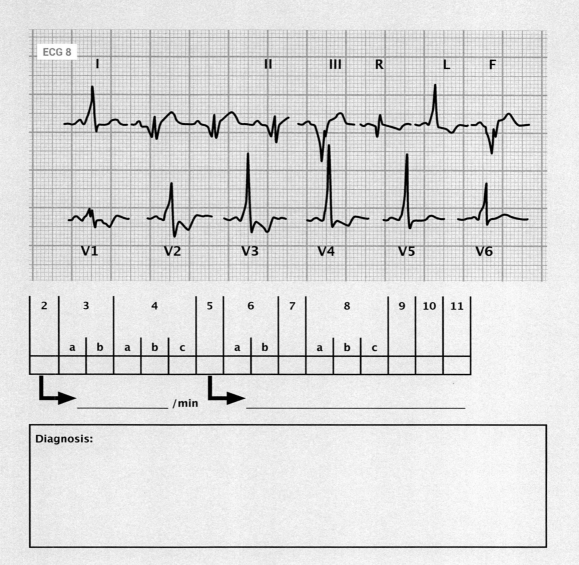

I   II   III   R   L   F

V1   V2   V3   V4   V5   V6

2	3		4			5	6	7	8			9	10	11
	a	b	a	b	c		a	b	a	b	c			

_____ /min   _____

Diagnosis:

Rhythm 101—the sinus rhythm

"To learn something new, take the path that you took yesterday."
—John Burroughs

Rhythm 101–the sinus rhythm

If you want to be able to diagnose rhythm problems, you'll first have to learn what constitutes a sinus rhythm (the healthy heart's normal rhythm). In sinus rhythm there's a regular sequence of P waves and QRS complexes.

Criteria for sinus rhythm

All of the following four criteria need to be met in order for sinus rhythm to be present: **(1)** P waves are positive in leads I and II; **(2)** every P wave is followed by a QRS complex; **(3)** the distance between each P wave and the following QRS is constant; and **(4)** the distance between the QRS complexes is constant. Let's check the example below for the presence of sinus rhythm.

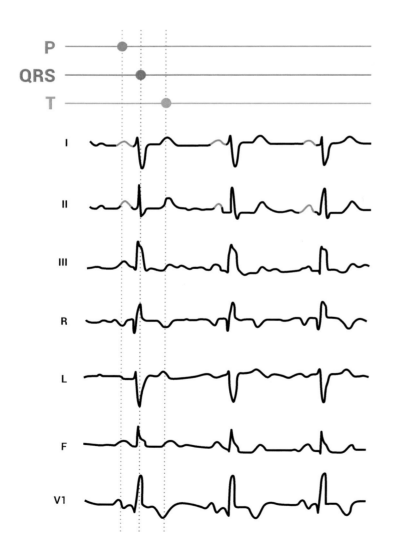

Sinus rhythm is present if the following criteria are met:

1. P waves are positive in leads I and II ✓
2. Every P wave is followed by a QRS complex ✓
3. The distance between each P wave and the following QRS complex is constant ✓
4. The distance between the QRS complexes is constant ✓

↓

Sinus Rhythm

Note that apart from the limb leads, we also show you lead V1 here. This lead is located in close proximity to the right atrium and is therefore ideally suited for the assessment of atrial depolarization. The P wave is usually biphasic in lead V1, the initial positive deflection corresponds to right atrial depolarization, and the second (negative) part corresponds to left atrial depolarization.

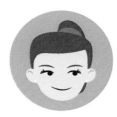

We have now covered all the steps of the cookbook! You're almost done with the final level. You are now able to speak the ECG language. You understand the most important principles and are able to carry out a basic evaluation of the ECG. Great job!

Question	Answer	Diagnosis
1. Rhythm	Criteria for sinus rhythm: 1. Are the P waves positive in I and II? 2. Is there a QRS complex after each P wave? 3. Are the PR intervals constant? 4. Are the RR intervals constant?	sinus rhythm or no sinus rhythm?
2. Heart rate	Estimate heart rate: 300/number of large boxes between two QRS complexes	heart rate in beats per min
3. P waves	a) Large P-wave amplitude (>2.5 mm in II, III, or aVF)	right atrial enlargement
	b) Prolonged negative part of P wave in V1 (1 mm) and P wave with 2 peaks in II, P-wave duration >0.12 s	left atrial enlargement
4. PR interval	a) >0.2 s (if PR interval constant for all beats and each P wave is followed by a QRS complex)	I° AV block
	b) <0.12 s and QRS complex normal	LGL syndrome
	c) <0.12 s and visible delta wave	WPW syndrome
5. QRS axis	Determine the axis according to leads I, II, and aVF	normal axis left axis deviation right axis deviation northwest axis
6. QRS duration	a) ≥0.12 s (always think of WPW syndrome as a differential)	complete bundle branch block
	b) >0.1 s and <0.12 s with typical bundle branch block appearance (notching)	incomplete bundle branch block
7. Rotation	Rotation is defined according to the heart's transition zone. Normally the transition zone is located at V4, which means that right ventricular myocardium is located at V1–V3 and left ventricular myocardium is at V5–V6.	transition zone at V5–V6: clockwise rotation transition zone at V1–V3: counterclockwise rotation NOTE: don't evaluate rotation in the setting of myocardial infarction, WPW syndrome, or bundle branch block
8. QRS amplitude	a) QRS amplitude <0.5 mV in all standard leads	low voltage
	b) Positive criteria for left ventricular hypertrophy	left ventricular hypertrophy
	c) Positive criteria for right ventricular hypertrophy	right ventricular hypertrophy
9. QRS infarction signs	abnormal Q waves, QS waves, missing R-wave progression	myocardial infarction; localization according to affected leads

10. ST–T segment

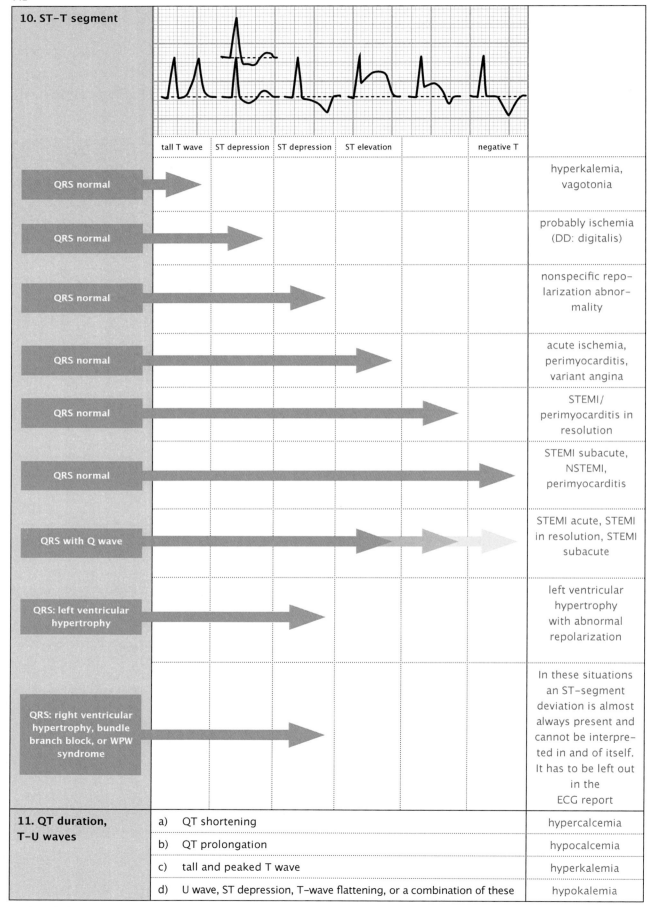

	tall T wave	ST depression	ST depression	ST elevation		negative T	
QRS normal	→						hyperkalemia, vagotonia
QRS normal		→					probably ischemia (DD: digitalis)
QRS normal			→				nonspecific repolarization abnormality
QRS normal				→			acute ischemia, perimyocarditis, variant angina
QRS normal					→		STEMI/ perimyocarditis in resolution
QRS normal						→	STEMI subacute, NSTEMI, perimyocarditis
QRS with Q wave				→ → →			STEMI acute, STEMI in resolution, STEMI subacute
QRS: left ventricular hypertrophy			→				left ventricular hypertrophy with abnormal repolarization
QRS: right ventricular hypertrophy, bundle branch block, or WPW syndrome			→				In these situations an ST–segment deviation is almost always present and cannot be interpreted in and of itself. It has to be left out in the ECG report

11. QT duration, T–U waves			
	a)	QT shortening	hypercalcemia
	b)	QT prolongation	hypocalcemia
	c)	tall and peaked T wave	hyperkalemia
	d)	U wave, ST depression, T-wave flattening, or a combination of these	hypokalemia

Level 13

QUIZ SECTION

Start by marking the P waves and the QRS complexes, then decide whether sinus rhythm is present or not. Determine the heart rate in each example.

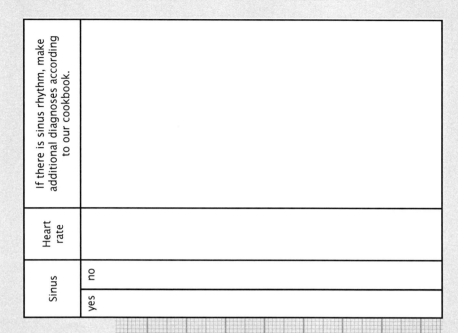

If there is sinus rhythm, make additional diagnoses according to our cookbook.	
Heart rate	
Sinus	no
	yes

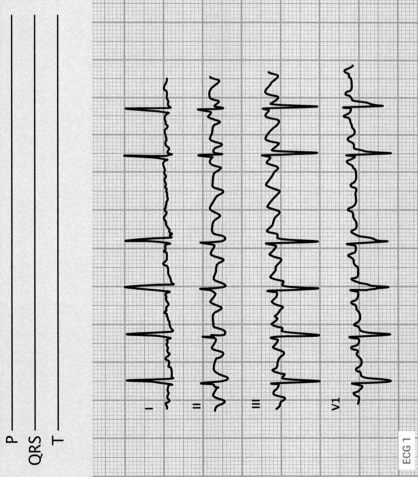

P
QRS
T

I

II

III

V1

ECG 1

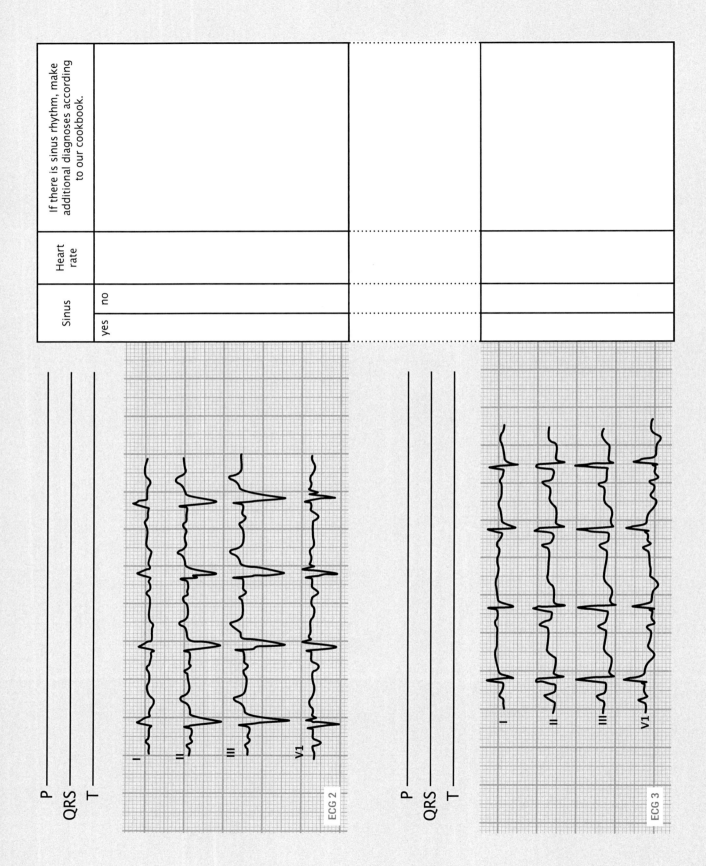

Sinus		Heart rate	If there is sinus rhythm, make additional diagnoses according to our cookbook.
	no		
	yes		

P

QRS

T

ECG 2

P

QRS

T

ECG 3

Sinus		Heart rate	If there is sinus rhythm, make additional diagnoses according to our cookbook.
	no		
yes			

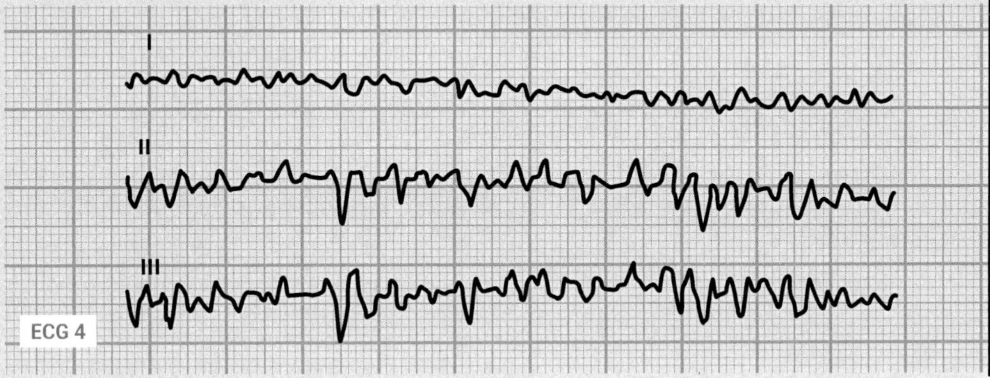

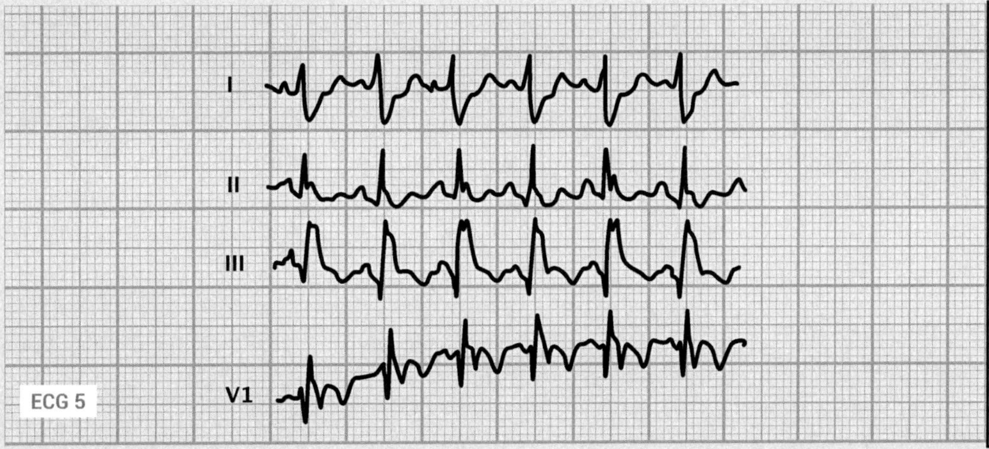

P _____

QRS _____

T _____

ECG 4

I

II

III

P _____

QRS _____

T _____

ECG 5

I

II

III

v1

Sinus		Heart rate	If there is sinus rhythm, make additional diagnoses according to our cookbook.
	no		
yes			

P _____

QRS _____

T _____

I

II

III

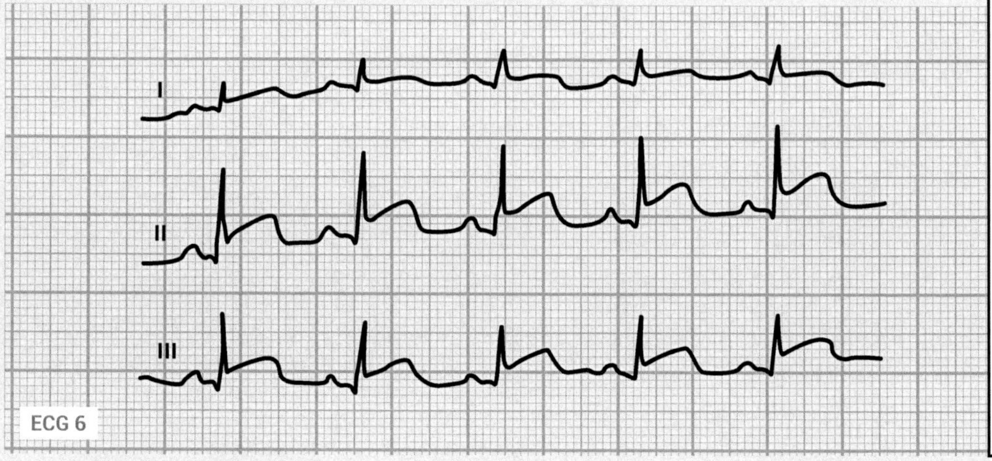

ECG 6

Sinus		Heart rate	If there is sinus rhythm, make additional diagnoses according to our cookbook.
	no		
yes			

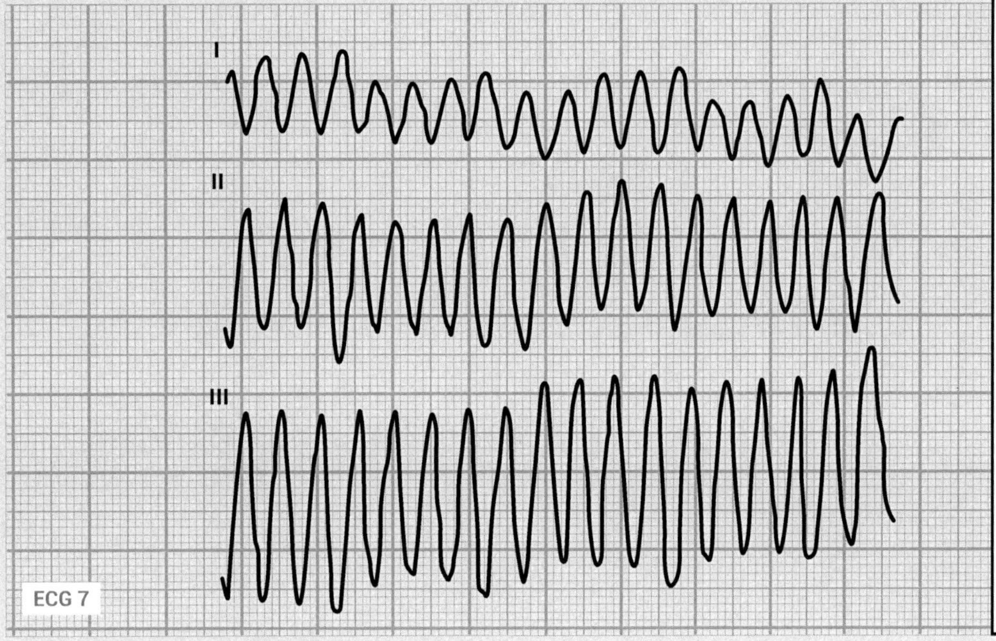

P _____

QRS _____

T _____

I

II

III

ECG 7

Sinus		Heart rate	If there is sinus rhythm, make additional diagnoses according to our cookbook.
yes	no		

P
QRS
T

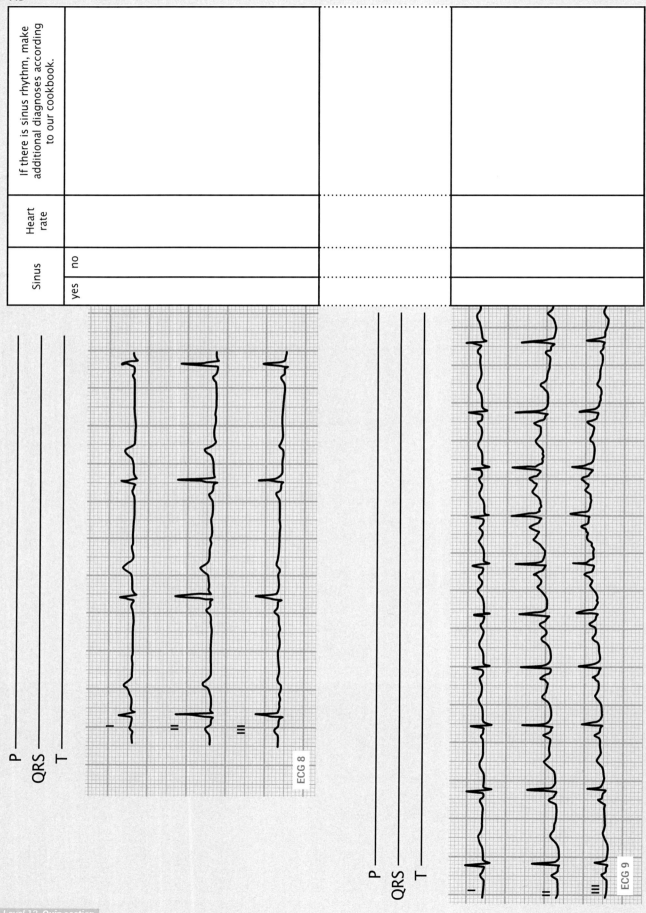

I

II

III

ECG 8

P
QRS
T

I

II

III

ECG 9

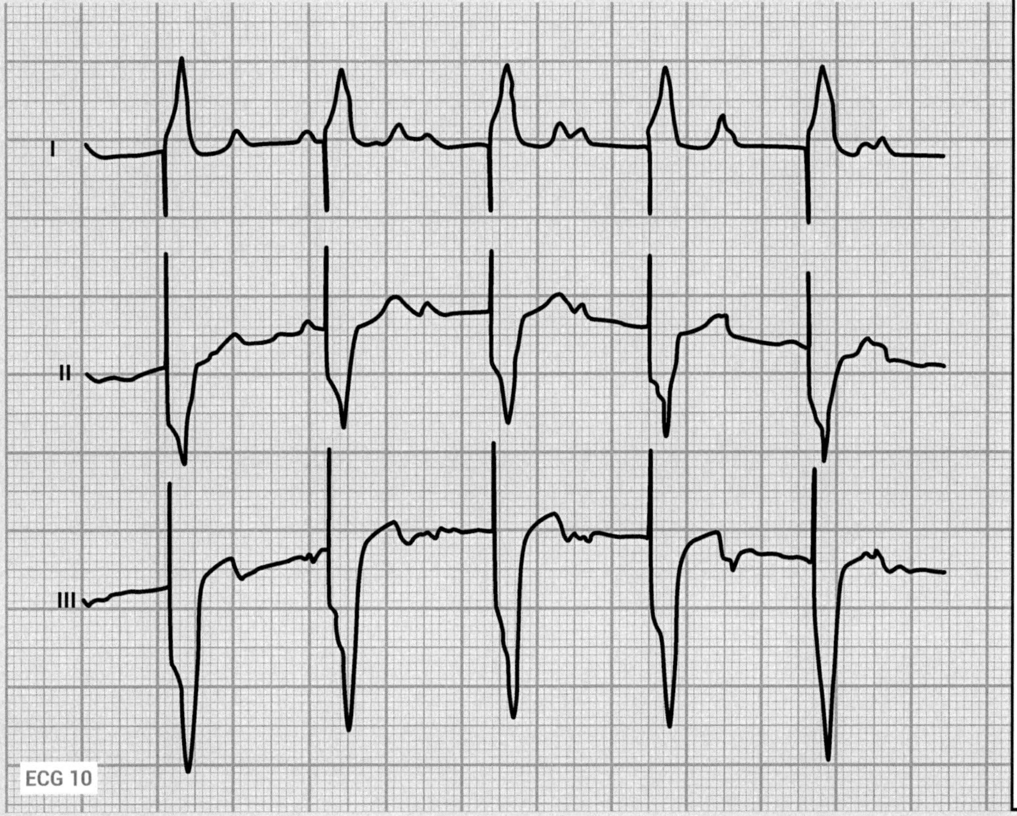

Sinus	Heart rate	If there is sinus rhythm, make additional diagnoses according to our cookbook.
yes / no		

P

QRS

T

I

II

III

ECG 10

Quiz Solutions

QUIZ SOLUTION

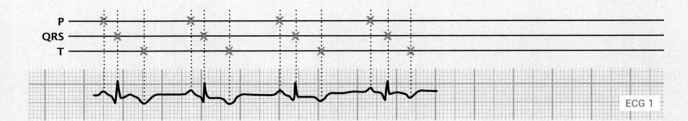

This is an easy example, as P waves, QRS complexes, and T waves follow each other in a regular fashion.

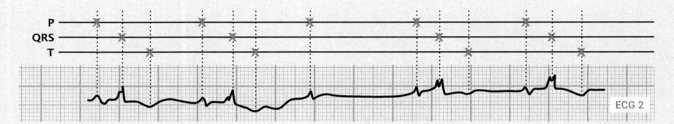

As this is a more difficult example, use the technique of looking for the sharpest wave in order to identify the QRS complexes (4 QRS complexes can be found in this example). The T wave appears 5–10 mm behind each QRS complex. The remaining 5 waves are not as sharp as the QRS complex, but are sharper than the T wave and therefore must be P waves.

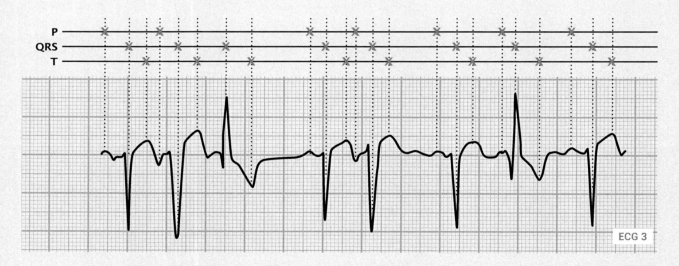

It is important to note that the QRS complexes show 3 different morphologies in this example. However, they can be identified as the sharpest waves. Furthermore, the T waves can be found 5–10 mm after each QRS complex. The P waves are not uniform and most are positive, but the 2nd and the 4th P waves are negative.

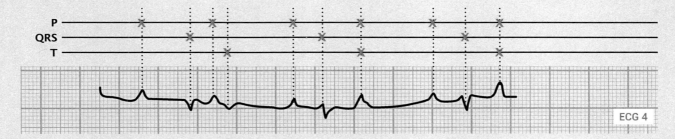

ECG 4

What makes this ECG a little bit tricky is the fact that P and QRS amplitudes are almost the same. However, the QRS complexes have sharper edges than the P waves. Also, P and T waves interfere with one another at some occasions (e.g., the 4th and the 6th P waves). Remember that the P waves usually occur at very regular intervals. We should therefore be able to predict where the next P wave should appear (this also applies to examples 1 and 2 above).

QUIZ SOLUTION

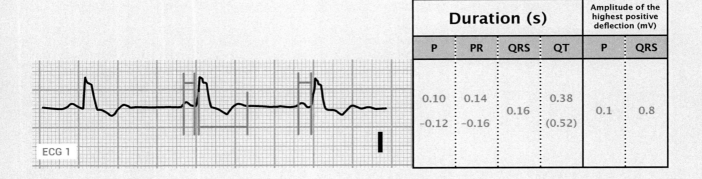

ECG 1

Duration (s)				Amplitude of the highest positive deflection (mV)	
P	PR	QRS	QT	P	QRS
0.10	0.14	0.16	0.38	0.1	0.8
-0.12	-0.16		(0.52)		

As the P wave does not start and end with a sharp deflection but deviates from the isoelectric line rather smoothly, it can sometimes be hard to measure its exact duration. You may get different results depending on which P wave you are measuring (e.g., 2nd P wave 0.1 s, 3rd P wave 0.12 s). If in doubt, you should perform the measurements in different leads. The same applies to the QT interval—the end of the T wave is sometimes hard to determine. Whether the positive deflection at the end was interpreted as a U wave or as part of a biphasic T wave makes a big difference (0.38 or 0.52 s). So always have a look at several leads when performing tricky measurements!

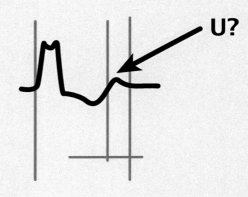

U?

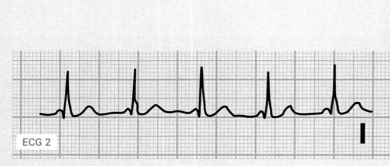

ECG 2

Duration (s)				Amplitude of the highest positive deflection (mV)	
P	PR	QRS	QT	P	QRS
0.08	0.08	0.08	0.36	0.15	1.3

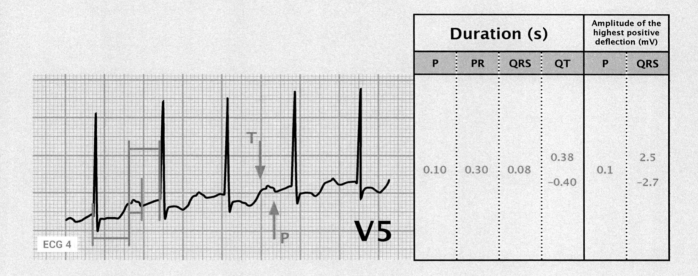

Duration (s)				Amplitude of the highest positive deflection (mV)	
P	PR	QRS	QT	P	QRS
0.08	0.08	0.12	0.44 -0.48	0.1	1.1

ECG 3

Also in this example, the end of the T wave is difficult to determine.

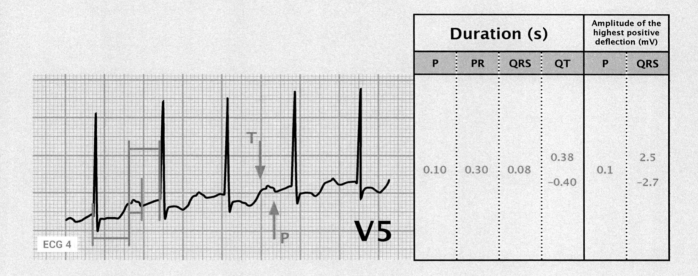

Duration (s)				Amplitude of the highest positive deflection (mV)	
P	PR	QRS	QT	P	QRS
0.10	0.30	0.08	0.38 -0.40	0.1	2.5 -2.7

ECG 4   V5

This example is difficult because of the close proximity of the T and P waves. Look at the second beat—the vertical line marks the beginning of the next P wave and the end of the preceding T wave. We need this information in order to determine the QT duration (of the 1st beat). The amplitude of the QRS complex in the 5 beats of this example varies between 2.5 and 2.7 mV. Such variation is common and usually reflects changes in the heart's position due to breathing.

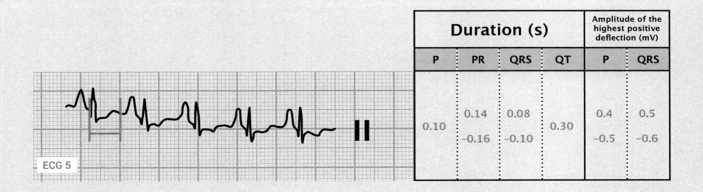

Duration (s)				Amplitude of the highest positive deflection (mV)	
P	PR	QRS	QT	P	QRS
0.10	0.14 -0.16	0.08 -0.10	0.30	0.4 -0.5	0.5 -0.6

ECG 5

156

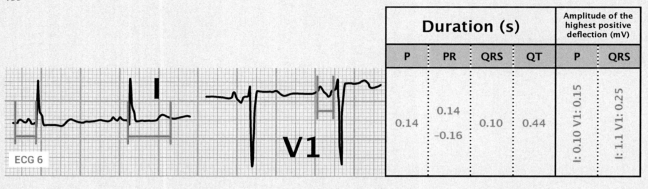

Duration (s)				Amplitude of the highest positive deflection (mV)	
P	PR	QRS	QT	P	QRS
0.14	0.14 −0.16	0.10	0.44	I: 0.10 V1: 0.15	I: 1.1 V1: 0.25

ECG 6

The different time intervals (e.g., PR interval, QRS duration, QT interval) should be the same in all the leads of the same ECG. For example, the P wave measures 0.14 s in lead I as well as in V1. The amplitudes of the different waves of the ECG, however, vary greatly from lead to lead. Just have a look at the R wave of 1.1 mV in lead I and compare that to the R wave amplitude of 0.25 mV in V1.

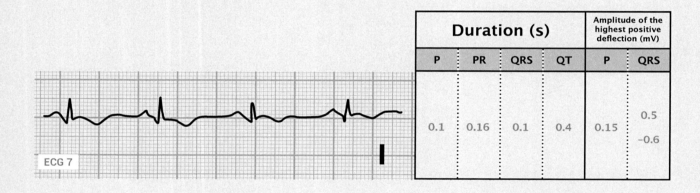

Duration (s)				Amplitude of the highest positive deflection (mV)	
P	PR	QRS	QT	P	QRS
0.1	0.16	0.1	0.4	0.15	0.5 −0.6

ECG 7

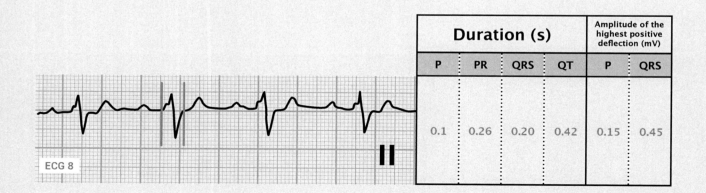

Duration (s)				Amplitude of the highest positive deflection (mV)	
P	PR	QRS	QT	P	QRS
0.1	0.26	0.20	0.42	0.15	0.45

ECG 8

Level 3

QUIZ SOLUTION

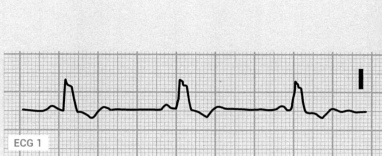

P mitrale	I° AV block	LGL syndrome	WPW syndrome	Complete bundle branch block	None of the answers provided
				x	

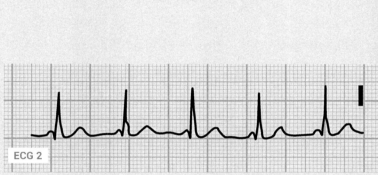

P mitrale	I° AV block	LGL syndrome	WPW syndrome	Complete bundle branch block	None of the answers provided
		x			

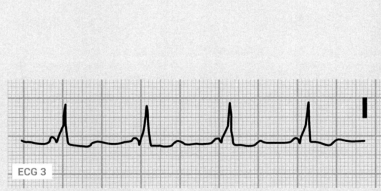

P mitrale	I° AV block	LGL syndrome	WPW syndrome	Complete bundle branch block	None of the answers provided
			x		

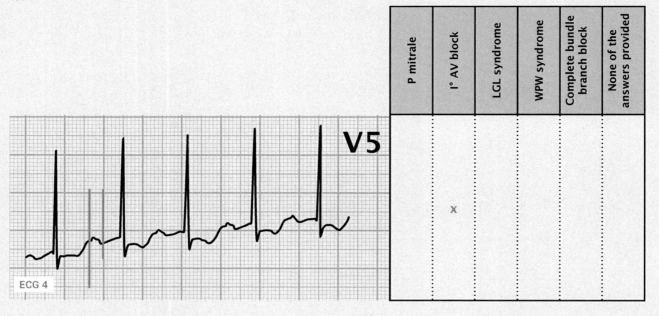

	P mitrale	I° AV block	LGL syndrome	WPW syndrome	Complete bundle branch block	None of the answers provided
ECG 4		x				

At first glance, especially looking at the third beat, one may suspect the presence of a P mitrale. The P wave seems to be double-peaked with a length of 0.16 s. However, when looking at the first beat, you'll notice the fusion of the T and P waves. We added two vertical lines to the ECG. The first one indicates the end of the T wave and the start of the following P wave. The second one indicates the end of the P wave. So the P wave itself is not double-peaked, nor is it prolonged. On the other hand, the PR interval is clearly lengthened, which indicates the presence of first degree AV block.

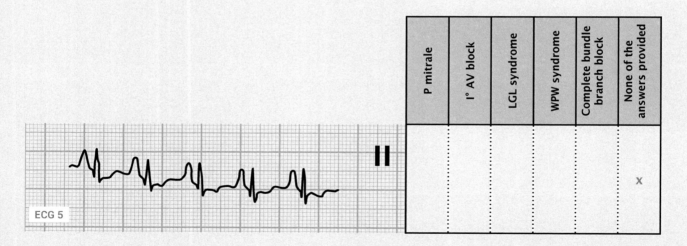

	P mitrale	I° AV block	LGL syndrome	WPW syndrome	Complete bundle branch block	None of the answers provided
ECG 5						x

In this example, none of the suggested options is correct. You have certainly noticed that the P waves are very sharp and exceptionally high (0.5 mV). As you will learn later, this may be due to right atrial hypertrophy.

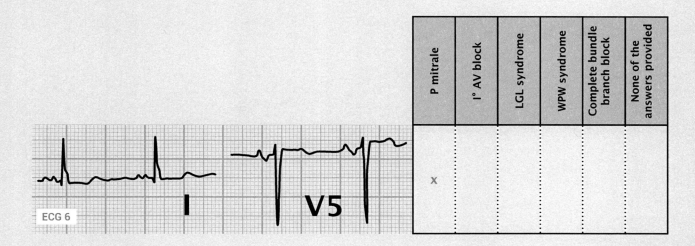

	P mitrale	I° AV block	LGL syndrome	WPW syndrome	Complete bundle branch block	None of the answers provided
ECG 6	x					

The P wave in this example is double-peaked and longer than normal (0.14 s in lead I). This is a typical case of P mitrale resulting from volume overload and dilatation of the left atrium.

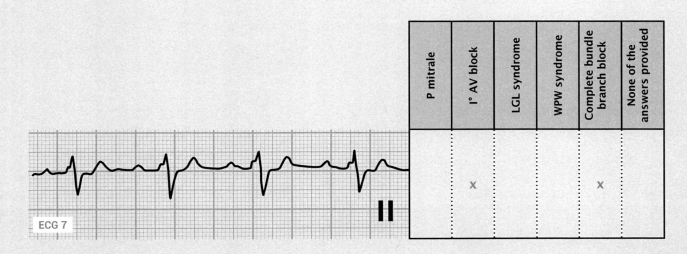

	P mitrale	I° AV block	LGL syndrome	WPW syndrome	Complete bundle branch block	None of the answers provided
ECG 7		x			x	

In this example we can see a prolonged QRS complex (bundle branch block) and a prolonged PR duration (first degree AV block).

QUIZ SOLUTION

Which leads provide information on the...	V1	V2	V3	V4	V5	V6	V7	V8
Right ventricle	X	X	X					
Upper part of the septum		X	X					
Left ventricle		X	X	X	X	X	X	X
Anterior wall of the LV		X	X	X				
Lateral wall of the LV					X	X		
Posterior wall of the LV							X	X

Which ventricle is represented by these leads under normal circumstances?

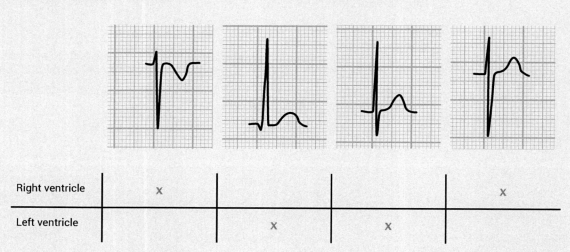

Right ventricle	X			X
Left ventricle		X	X	

QUIZ SOLUTION

These examples demonstrate one important pheno-menon: in bundle branch block, depolarization and repolarization show in opposite directions. What does that mean? Well, in right bundle branch block, the QRS complexes in leads V1 and V2 are mainly positive but the T waves are usually negative. And in left bundle branch block, the QRS complexes in V5 and V6 are mainly positive, while the T waves in these same leads are negative. This is true for examples 1, 2, 3, and 5. If you take a closer look at example 3, you'll see that T waves are also negative in leads V5 and V6, which cannot be attributed to right bundle branch block. So there must be some other cause for this repolarization problem, like, for example, coronary artery disease.

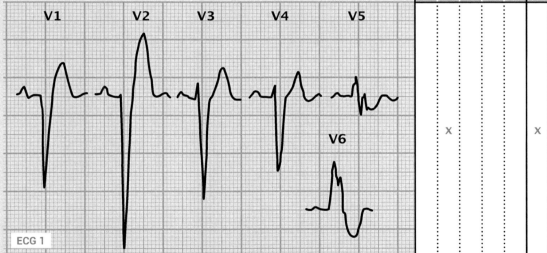

ECG 1

Diagnosis					Diagnostic criteria				
Complete right bundle branch block	Complete left bundle branch block	Volume overload right ventricle	Volume overload left ventricle	WPW syndrome	Duration of the QRS complex	(V1) QRS shape	(V6) QRS shape	Duration of the PR interval	Delta wave in leads:
X					X	X			

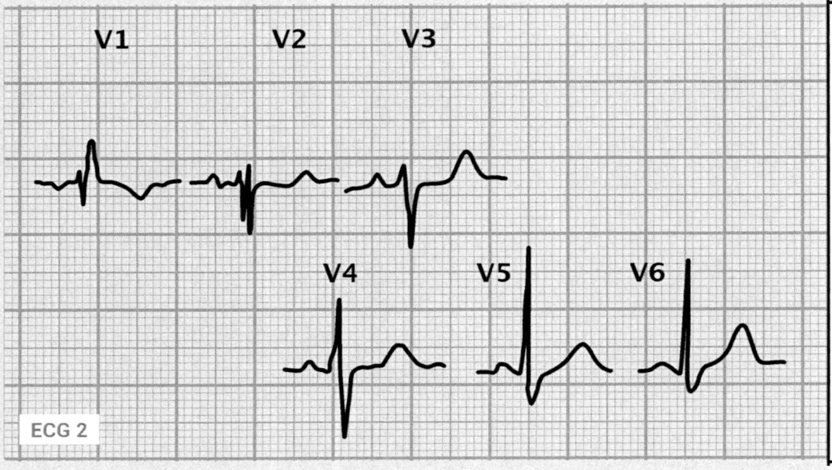

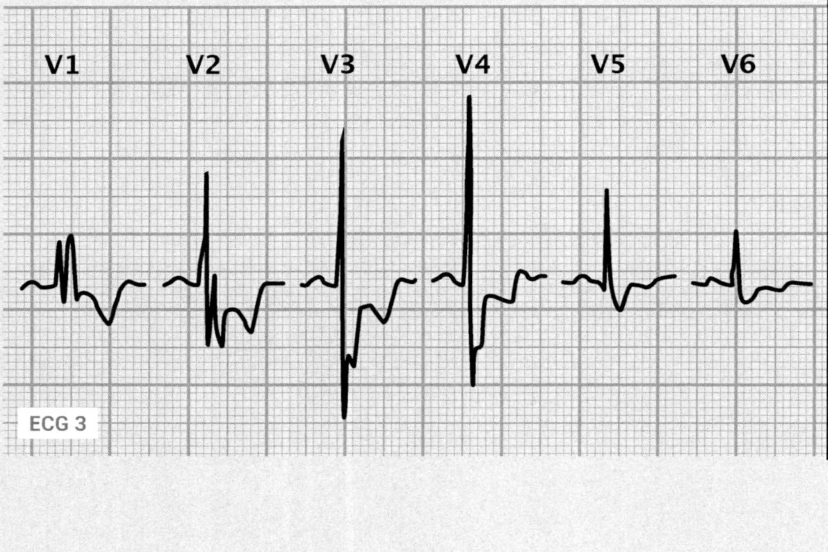

ECG 2

ECG 3

	Diagnosis					Diagnostic criteria				
	Complete right bundle branch block	Complete left bundle branch block	Volume overload right ventricle	Volume overload left ventricle	WPW syndrome	Duration of the QRS complex	(V1) QRS shape	(V6) QRS shape	Duration of the PR interval	Delta wave in leads:
ECG 2	X					X	X			
ECG 3	X					X	X			

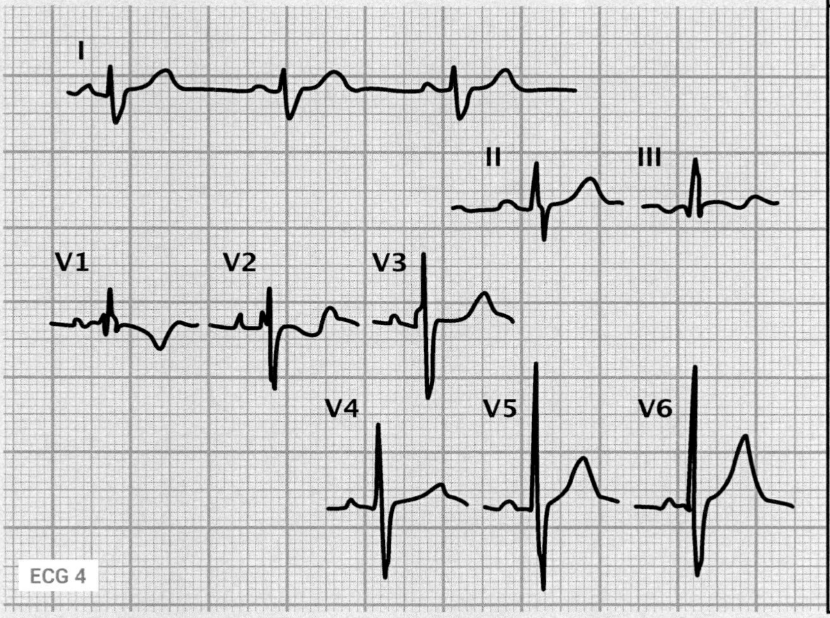

	Diagnosis					Diagnostic criteria				
Complete right bundle branch block	Complete left bundle branch block	Volume overload right ventricle	Volume overload left ventricle	WPW syndrome		Duration of the QRS complex	(V1) QRS shape	(V6) QRS shape	Duration of the PR interval	Delta wave in leads:
						x				

ECG 4

The notching of the QRS complex seen in lead V1 is called a right ventricular conduction delay. This RV conduction delay may be a normal finding in young healthy individuals (under the age of 20 years).

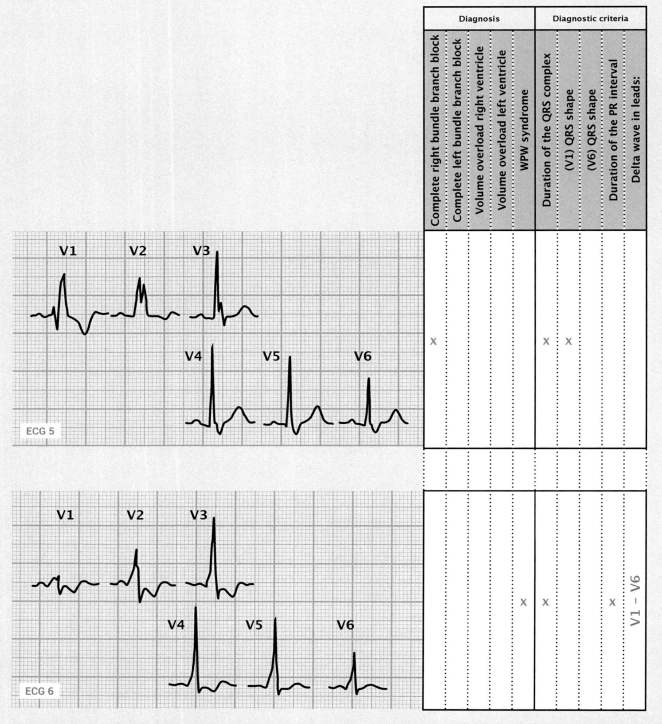

	Diagnosis					Diagnostic criteria				
	Complete right bundle branch block	Complete left bundle branch block	Volume overload right ventricle	Volume overload left ventricle	WPW syndrome	Duration of the QRS complex	(V1) QRS shape	(V6) QRS shape	Duration of the PR interval	Delta wave in leads:
ECG 5	X					X	X			
ECG 6					X	X			X	V1 – V6

The broad and notched QRS complex in V1 may be misinterpreted as right bundle branch block. When in fact, the first R wave corresponds to the delta wave, which can be even more clearly appreciated from V2 onward.

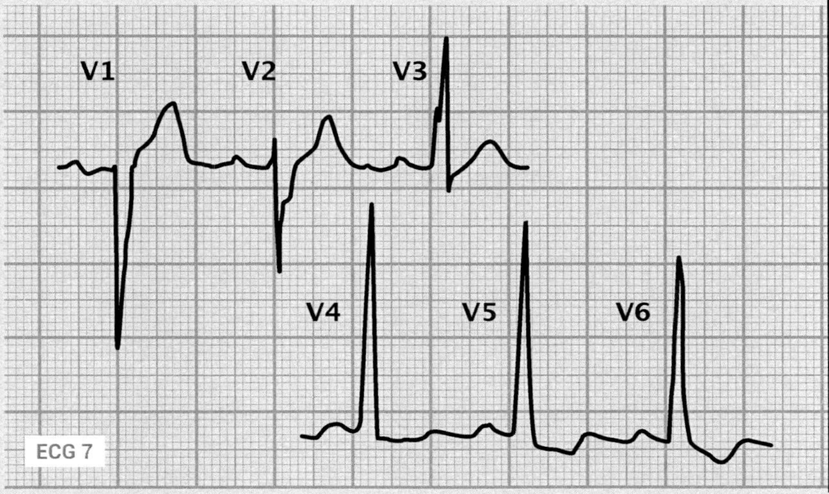

ECG 7

	Diagnosis					Diagnostic criteria				
Complete right bundle branch block	Complete left bundle branch block	Volume overload right ventricle	Volume overload left ventricle	WPW syndrome		Duration of the QRS complex	(V1) QRS shape	(V6) QRS shape	Duration of the PR interval	Delta wave in leads:
				x		x	x			

QUIZ SOLUTION

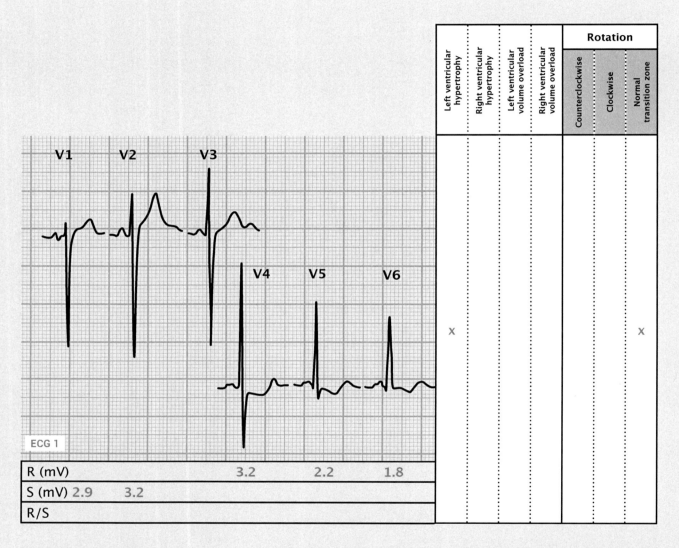

	Left ventricular hypertrophy	Right ventricular hypertrophy	Left ventricular volume overload	Right ventricular volume overload	Rotation		
					Counterclockwise	Clockwise	Normal transition zone
	X						X
R (mV)			3.2	2.2	1.8		
S (mV)	2.9	3.2					
R/S							

ECG 1

Calculation of the Sokolow index suggests that left ventricular hypertrophy is present (SV1 + RV5 = 5.1 mV, SV2 + RV6 = 5 mV, SV1 + RV6 = 4.7 mV, SV2 + RV5 = 5.4 mV). Usually only the highest value will be used, in this case SV2 + RV5. Some authors propose using only SV2 + RV6 or SV1 + RV5, which leads to a lower sensitivity and a higher specificity. You should always try to confirm your suspicion of ventricular hypertrophy with echocardiography.

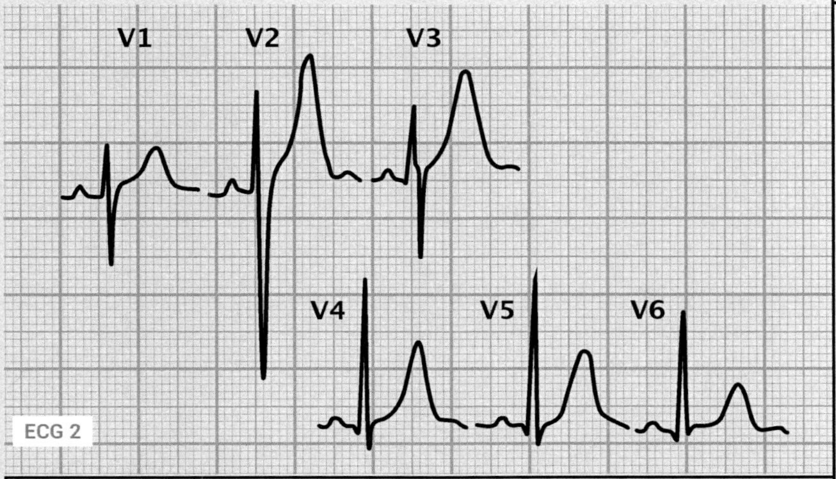

	Left ventricular hypertrophy	Right ventricular hypertrophy	Left ventricular volume overload	Right ventricular volume overload	Rotation		
					Counterclockwise	Clockwise	Normal transition zone
	X				X		X

R (mV)		1.9
S (mV)	2.4	
R/S		

V1 V2 V3

V4 V5 V6

ECG 2

High likelihood of left ventricular hypertrophy. The Sokolow index is 4.3 mV (SV2 + RV5 = 4.3 mV). This case shows that we cannot always make a clear-cut diagnosis of the transition zone. In V3 the S wave is still dominant, but in V4 the R wave is dominant, so the transition zone will be between V3 and V4. Thus it is a borderline case.

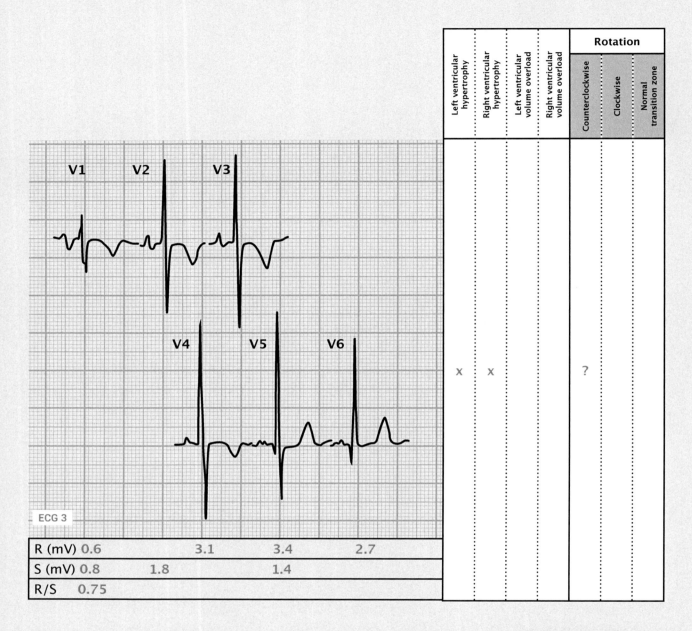

	Left ventricular hypertrophy	Right ventricular hypertrophy	Left ventricular volume overload	Right ventricular volume overload	Rotation		
					Counterclockwise	Clockwise	Normal transition zone
	x	x			?		

ECG 3

R (mV)	0.6		3.1	3.4	2.7
S (mV)	0.8	1.8		1.4	
R/S	0.75				

This is a rare example with signs of right and left ventricular hypertrophy: the high R/S ratio (0.75) along with a deep S wave in V5 suggests right ventricular hypertrophy. Also, the Sokolow index is positive, indicating left ventricular hypertrophy (SV2 + RV5 = 5.2 mV). So this is a case of biventricular hypertrophy. In this setting, diagnosis of rotation is not really possible.

The high R/S ratio in V1, together with a deep S wave in V5 and an M shape of the QRS complex in V1, suggests the presence of right ventricular hypertrophy.

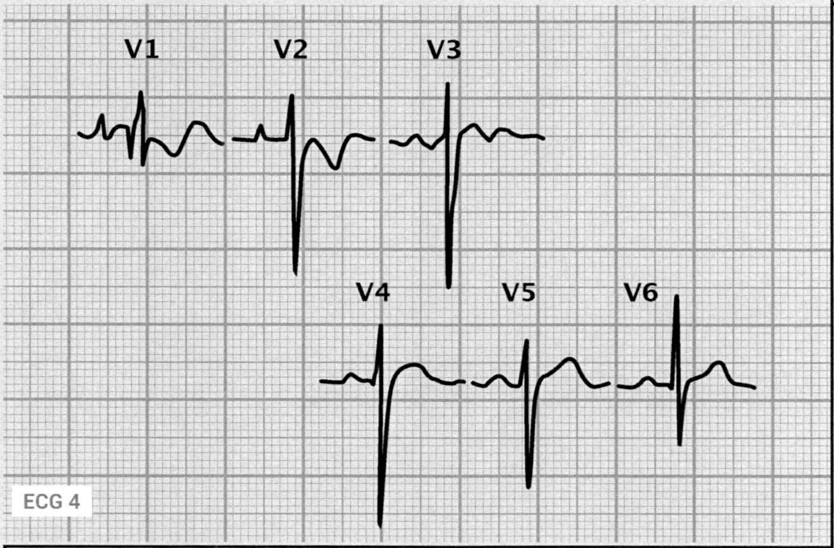

ECG 4

R (mV)	0.6		1.2
S (mV)	0.3	1.3	
R/S	2.0		

ECG 5

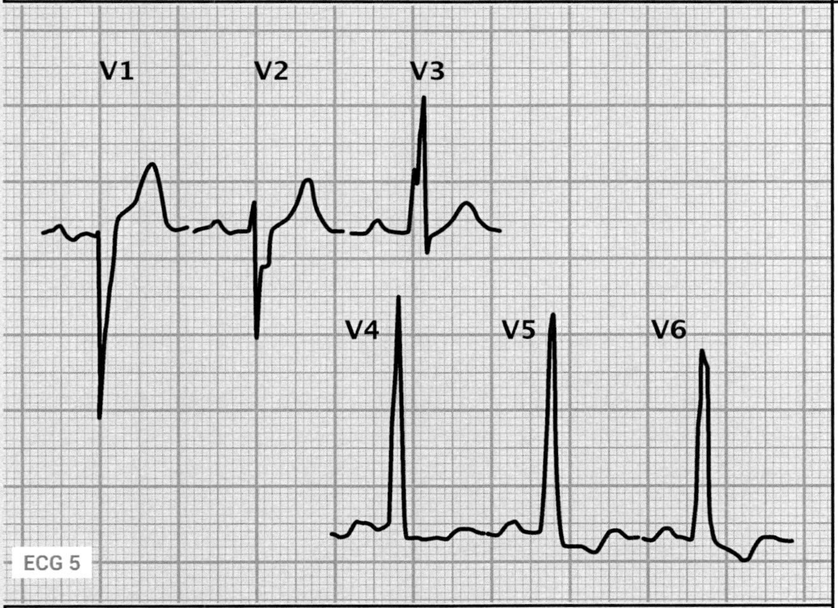

R (mV)	0.05	3.0	2.8	2.5
S (mV)	2.4			
R/S	0.02			

	Left ventricular hypertrophy	Right ventricular hypertrophy	Left ventricular volume overload	Right ventricular volume overload	Rotation		
					Counterclockwise	Clockwise	Normal transition zone
ECG 4		X		X		X	
ECG 5	X		X		X		

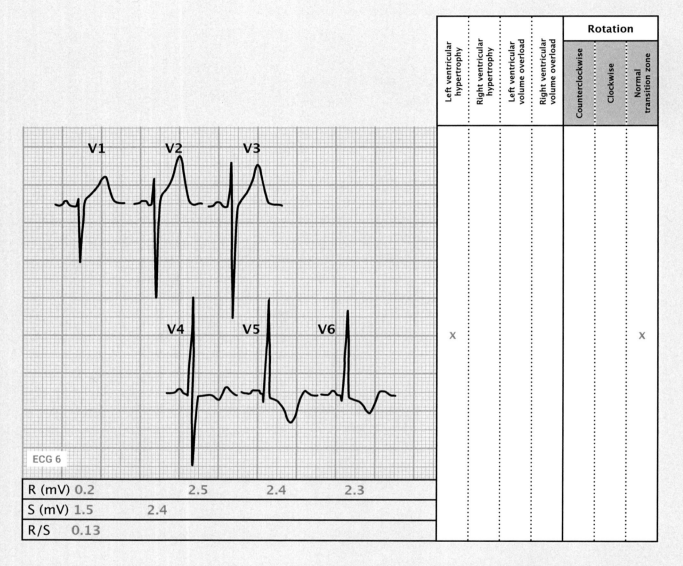

	Left ventricular hypertrophy	Right ventricular hypertrophy	Left ventricular volume overload	Right ventricular volume overload	Rotation		
					Counterclockwise	Clockwise	Normal transition zone
	X						X

R (mV)	0.2	2.5	2.4	2.3	
S (mV)	1.5	2.4			
R/S	0.13				

ECG 6

V1 V2 V3
V4 V5 V6

The Sokolow index (SV2 + RV5 = 4.8 mV) suggests left ventricular hypertrophy. Note that left ventricular hypertrophy may be associated with normal repolarization in the ECG (positive T waves in leads with more prominent R waves than S waves, as can be seen in examples 2 and 8). However, some patients with ventricular hypertrophy do have negative T waves, such as here.

	Left ventricular hypertrophy	Right ventricular hypertrophy	Left ventricular volume overload	Right ventricular volume overload	Rotation		
					Counterclockwise	Clockwise	Normal transition zone

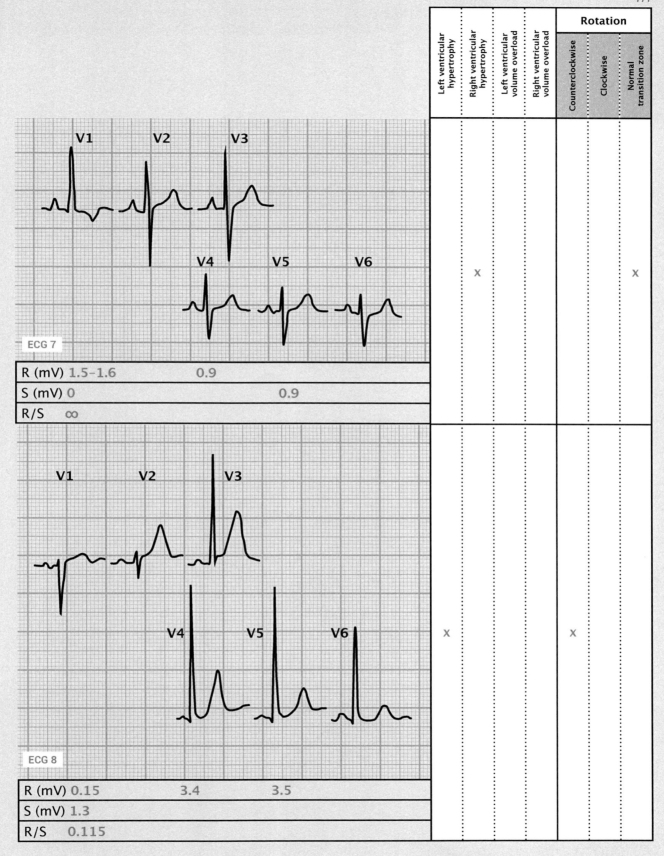

ECG 7

	X						X

R (mV)	1.5–1.6	0.9
S (mV)	0	0.9
R/S	∞	

ECG 8

	X				X		

R (mV)	0.15	3.4	3.5
S (mV)	1.3		
R/S	0.115		

The Sokolow index suggests left ventricular hypertrophy. Furthermore, counterclockwise rotation is also present in this patient.

QUIZ SOLUTION

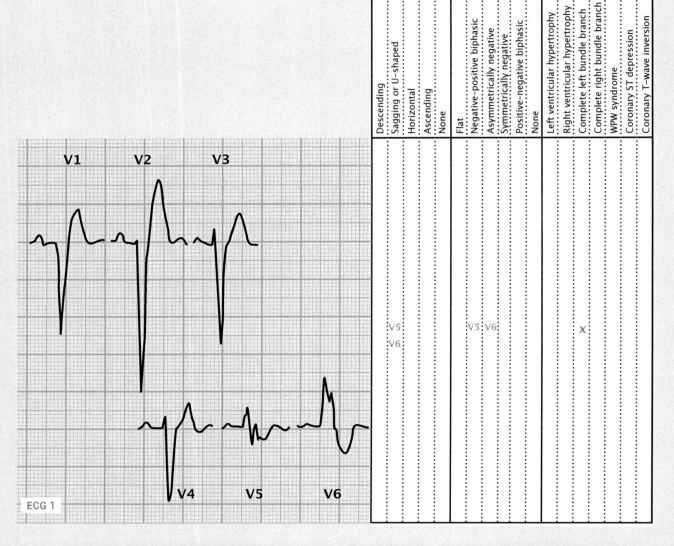

ST depression					T negativity						Diagnosis						
Descending	Sagging or U-shaped	Horizontal	Ascending	None	Flat	Negative–positive biphasic	Asymmetrically negative	Symmetrically negative	Positive–negative biphasic	None	Left ventricular hypertrophy	Right ventricular hypertrophy	Complete left bundle branch	Complete right bundle branch	WPW syndrome	Coronary ST depression	Coronary T-wave inversion
V5 V6					V5 V6								X				

ECG 1

A left bundle branch block is present (M shape in V5 and V6; QRS > 0.12 s). As expected in left bundle branch block, there are ST depressions and negative T waves in V5 and V6 as signs of impaired repolarization. The T wave is biphasic (negative–positive) in V5. Note that the ST depression over the left ventricle (V5, V6) is accompanied by an ST elevation in V1, V2 (mirror image). You can find similar changes in examples 2, 4, 5, and 7.

ST depression					T negativity						Diagnosis						
Descending	Sagging or U-shaped	Horizontal	Ascending	None	Flat	Negative–positive biphasic	Asymmetrically negative	Symmetrically negative	Positive–negative biphasic	None	Left ventricular hypertrophy	Right ventricular hypertrophy	Complete left bundle branch	Complete right bundle branch	WPW syndrome	Coronary ST depression	Coronary T-wave inversion
V5 V6							V5 V6				X						

Typical ECG changes associated with left ventricular hypertrophy: high R wave in V4, deep S wave in V1. Here we can use V4 for the calculation of the Sokolow index because the counterclockwise rotation of the heart (transition zone between V2 and V3) proves that V4 is definitely already left ventricle. The descending ST depressions and asymmetric T-wave inversions are signs of impaired repolarization in the setting of ventricular hypertrophy.

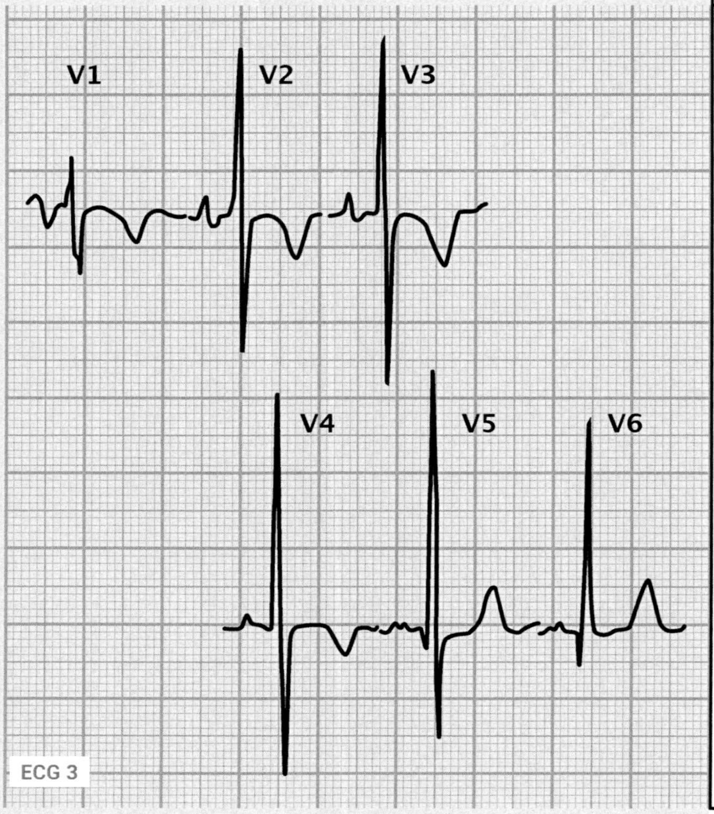

ECG 3

ST depression					T negativity						Diagnosis						
Descending	Sagging or U-shaped	Horizontal	Ascending	None	Flat	Negative-positive biphasic	Asymmetrically negative	Symmetrically negative	Positive-negative biphasic	None	Left ventricular hypertrophy	Right ventricular hypertrophy	Complete left bundle branch	Complete right bundle branch	WPW syndrome	Coronary ST depression	Coronary T-wave inversion
				x				V1 V2 V3 V4			x	x					

In this example, right ventricular hypertrophy (high R/S ratio in V1, deep S wave in V5) is present. Repolarization is impaired over the right ventricle (negative T waves in V1–V4). Left ventricular hypertrophy also seems to be present (positive Sokolow index). Repolarization over the left ventricle is normal.

The T waves in this example are normal although a bit flat in V5 and V6. Note the concave or horizontal ST depressions over the left ventricle, which could be a sign of coronary artery disease.

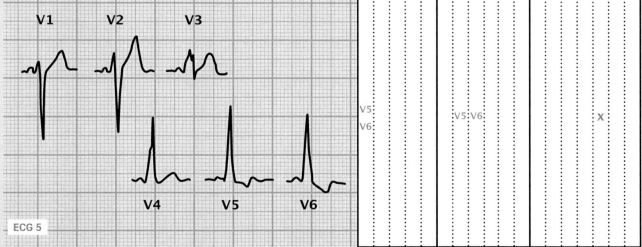

ECG 4

ST depression					T negativity						Diagnosis						
Descending	Sagging or U–shaped	Horizontal	Ascending	None	Flat	Negative–positive biphasic	Asymmetrically negative	Symmetrically negative	Positive–negative biphasic	None	Left ventricular hypertrophy	Right ventricular hypertrophy	Complete left bundle branch	Complete right bundle branch	WPW syndrome	Coronary ST depression	Coronary T–wave inversion
V5	V6	V4			X											X	

ECG 5

ST depression					T negativity						Diagnosis						
Descending	Sagging or U–shaped	Horizontal	Ascending	None	Flat	Negative–positive biphasic	Asymmetrically negative	Symmetrically negative	Positive–negative biphasic	None	Left ventricular hypertrophy	Right ventricular hypertrophy	Complete left bundle branch	Complete right bundle branch	WPW syndrome	Coronary ST depression	Coronary T–wave inversion
V5 V6					V5 V6										X		

There are several interesting findings in this ECG: ST elevation in V2, ST depression in V5 and V6, a short PR interval, and a slurred upstroke of the QRS complex. A delta wave is clearly visible in leads V3–V5. This is a case of WPW syndrome in which repolarization is almost always impaired.

These terminally negative biphasic T waves may be due to ACS or non-Q infarction in resolution. These changes can also be present in pericarditis.

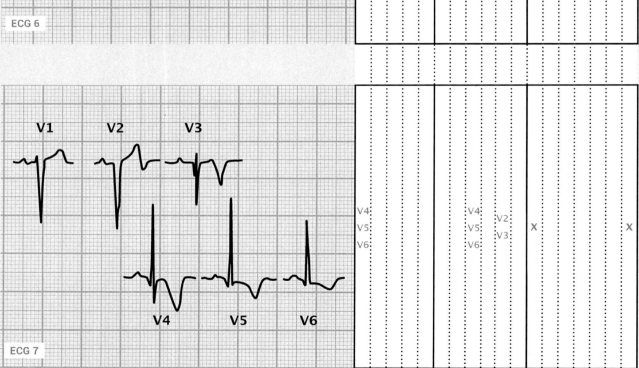

| ST depression | | | | | T negativity | | | | | | Diagnosis | | | | | | |
Descending	Sagging or U-shaped	Horizontal	Ascending	None	Flat	Negative–positive biphasic	Asymmetrically negative	Symmetrically negative	Positive–negative biphasic	None	Left ventricular hypertrophy	Right ventricular hypertrophy	Complete left bundle branch	Complete right bundle branch	WPW syndrome	Coronary ST depression	Coronary T–wave inversion
				X					V4 V5 V6								X

ECG 6

| ST depression | | | | | T negativity | | | | | | Diagnosis | | | | | | |
Descending	Sagging or U-shaped	Horizontal	Ascending	None	Flat	Negative–positive biphasic	Asymmetrically negative	Symmetrically negative	Positive–negative biphasic	None	Left ventricular hypertrophy	Right ventricular hypertrophy	Complete left bundle branch	Complete right bundle branch	WPW syndrome	Coronary ST depression	Coronary T–wave inversion
V4 V5 V6								V4 V5 V6	V2 V3		X						X

ECG 7

Left ventricular hypertrophy (positive Sokolow index) with accompanying ST-T wave changes in leads V5 and V6. Also, there's an old anteroseptal infarct (loss of R wave in V2 and Q wave in V3) with T-wave negativity in V2 and V3. So we have two different types of T-wave changes in this example—one due to left ventricular hypertrophy, the other one due to myocardial ischemia.

Level 8

QUIZ SOLUTION

Changes in QRS morphology related to myocardial infarction (pathologic Q wave, QS pattern, reduced initial R wave) can be found in leads								Infarction Localization						Which additional ECG changes can be found? (write them down)
V1	V2	V3	V4	V5	V6	V7	V8	Anteroseptal	Anterior wall	Lateral wall	Anterolateral region	Posterior wall	Posterolateral region	
X		X	(x)					X						First degree AV block, left ventricular hypertrophy

There's an R wave in V1, but in V2 it's missing. The QS morphology in V2 is compatible with an old anteroseptal infarct. The Q wave in V4 may be normal. As a consequence, the T waves are negative over the left ventricle. Furthermore the PR interval is prolonged to 0.28 s. First degree AV block is therefore present. The Sokolow index (SV1 + RV5 = 3.4 mV) is borderline, but the R wave in V4 alone exceeds 2.5 mV, so left ventricular hypertrophy becomes very probable.

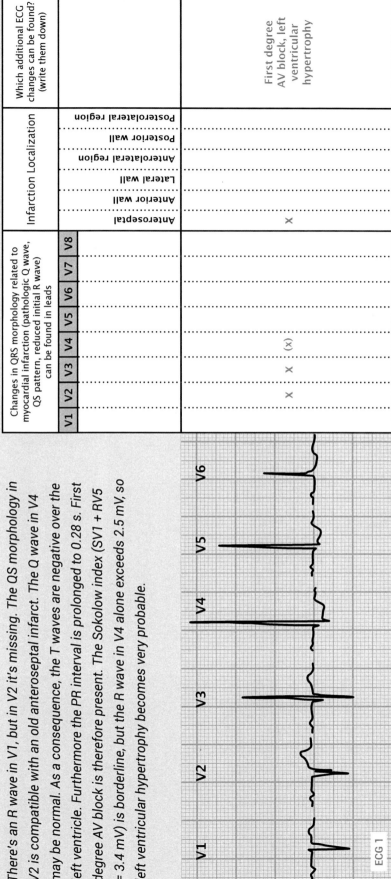

ECG 1

	Changes in QRS morphology related to myocardial infarction (pathologic Q wave, QS pattern, reduced initial R wave) can be found in leads								Infarction Localization						Which additional ECG changes can be found? (write them down)
	V1	V2	V3	V4	V5	V6	V7	V8	Anteroseptal	Anterior wall	Lateral wall	Anterolateral region	Posterior wall	Posterolateral region	
ECG 2				x	x	x						x			Complete right bundle branch block
ECG 3		x	x	(x)						x					acute phase

Note the Q waves (of 0.04 s) in V4–V6 suggesting anterolateral myocardial infarction. Also, the QRS complex is broadened to >0.12 s and has an M shape in V1. Right bundle branch block is therefore present.

ECG 2

The diagnosis in this case can be based on the loss of the initial R wave between V1 and V2. There is an R wave in V2, but it only appears after a Q wave and cannot be called an "initial R wave." The Q wave in V4 may be normal again. There is remarkable ST elevation in V2 and V3, and also slightly in V4, indicating the acute phase of the infarction.

ECG 3

Take a careful look at the Q waves in V5–V8. They appear small, but their amplitude has to be judged in comparison to the R waves of the same lead. Here the amplitude of the Q waves is as high as that of the R waves. Furthermore the duration of the Q waves (0.04 s) is significantly prolonged. Compared with the small amplitude of the QRS complex in V6, V7, and V8, the ST segment must also be considered to be elevated. This would classify the infarct as acute, which is strongly supported by the mirror image of ST depression in V2, V3, and V4.

Changes in QRS morphology related to myocardial infarction (pathologic Q wave, QS pattern, reduced initial R wave) can be found in leads								Infarction Localization						Which additional ECG changes can be found? (write them down)
V1	V2	V3	V4	V5	V6	V7	V8	Anteroseptal	Anterior wall	Lateral wall	Anterolateral region	Posterior wall	Posterolateral region	
					X	X	X						X	

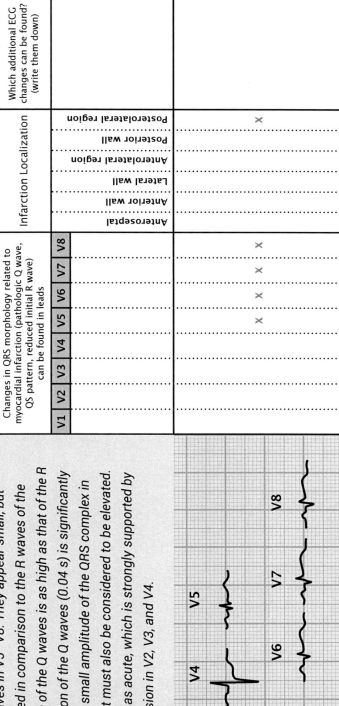

ECG 4

Changes in QRS morphology related to myocardial infarction (pathologic Q wave, QS pattern, reduced initial R wave) can be found in leads								Infarction Localization						Which additional ECG changes can be found? (write them down)
V1	V2	V3	V4	V5	V6	V7	V8	Anteroseptal	Anterior wall	Lateral wall	Anterolateral region	Posterior wall	Posterolateral region	
	X	X	X						X					Left ventricular hypertrophy
X	X	X	X	X							X			Complete right bundle branch block

The loss of the initial R wave (in V2), the negative T waves in V2 and V3, and the presence of a Q wave in V3 are signs of anteroseptal myocardial infarction. When we also consider the Q wave in V4 as pathologic (Q waves are decreasing from V4 to V6!), this would mean that the complete anterior wall is infarcted. The diagnosis of left ventricular hypertrophy is based on the Sokolow index (SV1 + RV5). The negative T waves over the left ventricle are a consequence of left ventricular hypertrophy.

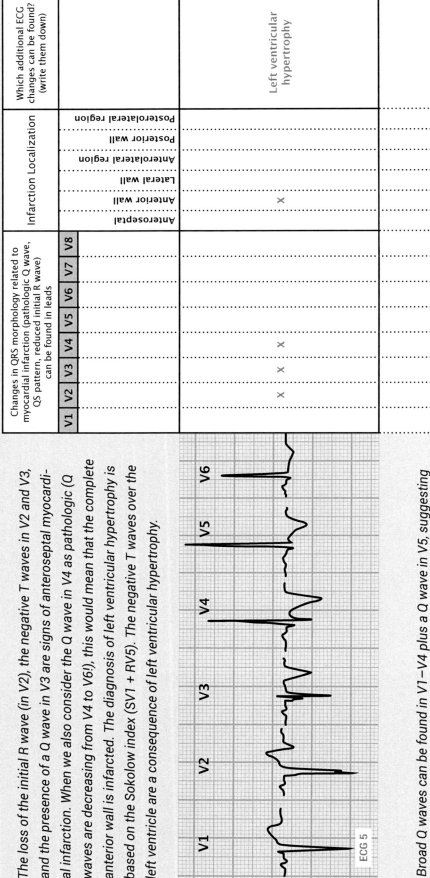

ECG 5

Broad Q waves can be found in V1–V4 plus a Q wave in V5, suggesting anterolateral myocardial infarction. Right bundle branch block is also present (QRS duration >0.12 s, M shape in V1).

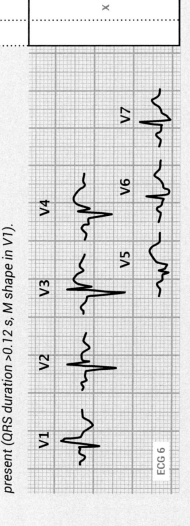

ECG 6

Level 9

QUIZ SOLUTION

Infarction	Inferior wall		X
	Posterior wall		
	Posterolateral region		?
	Lateral region		
	Anterolateral region		X
	Anterior wall		
	Anteroseptal region		
Hyper-trophy	Left ventricular hypertrophy		
	Right ventricular hypertrophy		
Rotation	Counterclockwise rotation	There is another pathology that won't allow me to evaluate rotation.	
	Clockwise rotation		
	Normal transition zone		
QRS duration	Dilated left ventricle		
	Dilated right ventricle		
	Complete LBBB		
	Complete RBBB		X
PR	LGL syndrome		
	WPW syndrome		
	I° AV block		

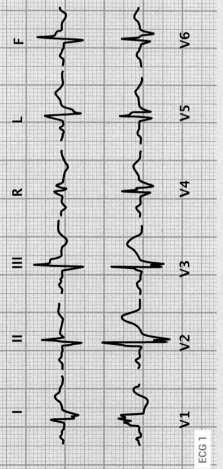

ECG 1

The QRS width is between 0.12 and 0.14 s, leading to the diagnosis of complete BBB. The QRS complex in V1 is M shaped, so this must be RBBB. Pathologic Q waves can be detected in leads II, III, and aVF as well as V4 to V6. So this must be an infarct of the inferior and lateral walls. If we also had V7 and V8 available, we might see Q waves there as well, which would indicate that the posterior wall was affected as well. The transitional zone in this example is located at V2 and V3, so we might suspect counterclockwise rotation. However, we have already learned that you cannot evaluate rotation in cases of BBB or myocardial infarction.

PR	I° AV block	
	WPW-syndrome	
	LGL-syndrome	
QRS duration	Complete RBBB	
	Complete LBBB	
	Dilated right ventricle	
	Dilated left ventricle	
Rotation	Normal transition zone	X
	Clockwise rotation	
	Counterclockwise rotation	
Hyper-trophy	Right ventricular hypertrophy	
	Left ventricular hypertrophy	X
Infarction	Anteroseptal region	
	Anterior wall	
	Anterolateral region	
	Lateral region	
	Posterolateral region	
	Posterior wall	
	Inferior wall	

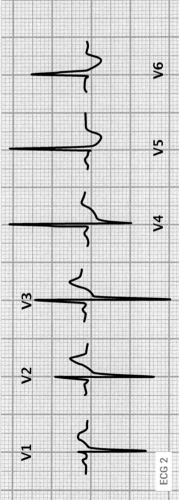

ECG 2

According to the Sokolow index, this must be left ventricular hypertrophy (with disturbed repolarization).

PR	I° AV block	
	WPW syndrome	
	LGL syndrome	
QRS duration	Complete RBBB	
	Complete LBBB	
	Dilated right ventricle	
	Dilated left ventricle	
Rotation	Normal transition zone	There's another pathology that won't allow me to evaluate rotation
	Clockwise rotation	
	Counterclockwise rotation	
Hyper-trophy	Right ventricular hypertrophy	
	Left ventricular hypertrophy	
Infarction	Anteroseptal region	
	Anterior wall	
	Anterolateral region	
	Lateral region	
	Posterolateral region	
	Posterior wall	
	Inferior wall	X

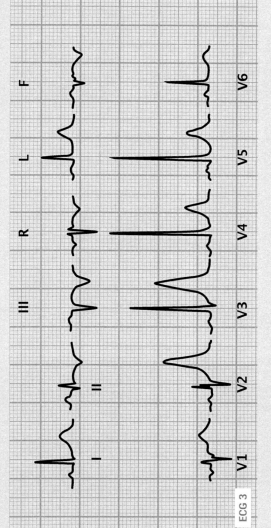

ECG 3

As we've already learned, you should not evaluate rotation in the setting of myocardial infarction. Note the very high T waves in leads V2 and V3, representing mirror images of T-wave inversions in leads II, III, and aVF.

PR	I° AV block	
	WPW syndrome	X
	LGL syndrome	
QRS duration	Complete RBBB	
	Complete LBBB	
	Dilated right ventricle	
	Dilated left ventricle	
Rotation	Normal transition zone	There's another pathology that won't allow me to evaluate rotation
	Clockwise rotation	
	Counterclockwise rotation	
Hyper-trophy	Right ventricular hypertrophy	
	Left ventricular hypertrophy	
Infarction	Anteroseptal region	
	Anterior wall	
	Anterolateral region	
	Lateral region	
	Posterolateral region	
	Posterior wall	
	Inferior wall	

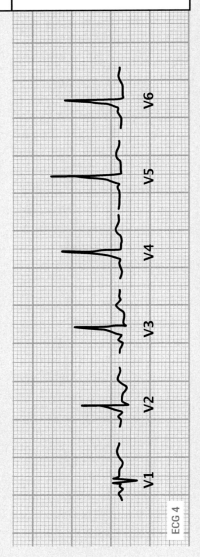

ECG 4

Making the diagnosis of WPW syndrome must be a piece of cake for you by now! This diagnosis does not allow statements of rotation, hypertrophy, infarction, etc.

Category	Finding	
PR	I° AV block	×
	WPW syndrome	
	LGL syndrome	
QRS duration	Complete RBBB	
	Complete LBBB	
	Dilated right ventricle	
	Dilated left ventricle	
Rotation	Normal transition zone	There's another pathology that won't allow me to evaluate rotation
	Clockwise rotation	
	Counterclockwise rotation	
Hyper-trophy	Right ventricular hypertrophy	
	Left ventricular hypertrophy	
Infarction	Anteroseptal region	
	Anterior wall	
	Anterolateral region	×
	Lateral region	
	Posterolateral region	
	Posterior wall	
	Inferior wall	×

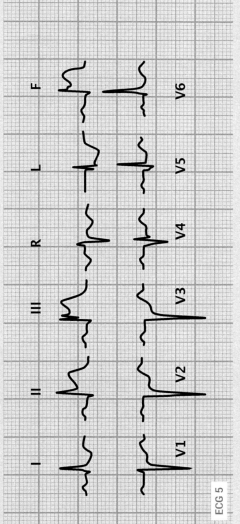

ECG 5

Changes in QRS morphology typical for myocardial infarction in the anteroseptal and lateral segments (QS in leads V2 and V3 and pathologic Q waves in leads V4 and V5). Furthermore, note the Q waves in leads I, II, III, aVL, and aVF. The Q waves in leads I and aVL represent lateral wall myocardial infarction, whereas the changes in leads II, III, and aVF indicate that the inferior wall also has a problem. You will learn later that the ST elevations in leads II, III, and aVF indicate the presence of acute inferior wall myocardial infarction.

QUIZ SOLUTION

In this example we cannot find changes in the QRS complex typical of myocardial infarction. On Feb 19, there were ST elevations in leads V2 to V5. On March 16, the ST segment has nearly returned to the isoelectric line and there remains a biphasic T wave in leads V4 to V6. There are two explanations for these changes: 1) perimyocarditis or 2) acute myocardial infarction without the subsequent development of Q waves. The extensive ST changes without the development of Q waves suggests an inflammatory cause. Finally, the patient was an 18-year-old male, which makes an acute coronary syndrome rather unlikely.

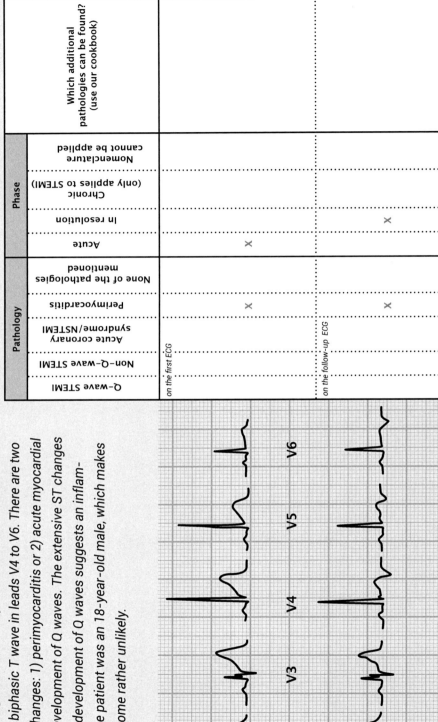

	Pathology					Phase				Which additional pathologies can be found? (use our cookbook)
	Q-wave STEMI	Non-Q-wave STEMI	Acute coronary syndrome/NSTEMI	Perimyocarditis	None of the pathologies mentioned	Acute	In resolution	Chronic (only applies to STEMI)	Nomenclature cannot be applied	
on the first ECG				X		X				
on the follow-up ECG				X			X			

Feb 19

V1 V2 V3 V4 V5 V6

March 16

ECG 1

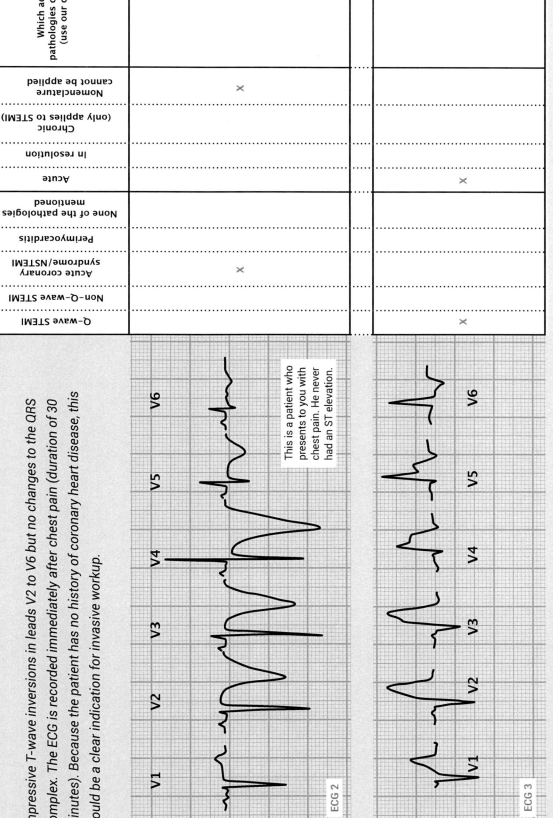

| Pathology | | | | | Phase | | | | Which additional pathologies can be found? (use our cookbook) |
Q-wave STEMI	Non-Q-wave STEMI	Acute coronary syndrome/NSTEMI	Perimyocarditis	None of the pathologies mentioned	Acute	In resolution	Chronic (only applies to STEMI)	Nomenclature cannot be applied	
		X						X	
X					X				

Impressive T-wave inversions in leads V2 to V6 but no changes to the QRS complex. The ECG is recorded immediately after chest pain (duration of 30 minutes). Because the patient has no history of coronary heart disease, this would be a clear indication for invasive workup.

V1 V2 V3 V4 V5 V6

This is a patient who presents to you with chest pain. He never had an ST elevation.

ECG 2

V1 V2 V3 V4 V5 V6

ECG 3

In addition to the acute ST-segment changes over the anterior wall, there are T-wave inversions in lead V6, suggesting preexisting repolarization problems in addition to the acute ischemic event.

Note the mirror images of an acute inferior ischemia in leads V2, V3, aVR, and aVL. The Q waves in leads II, III, and aVF are not deep and wide enough to make the diagnosis of Q-wave STEMI, but it is a typical pattern of acute ischemia, which may show Q waves within the next hour or so.

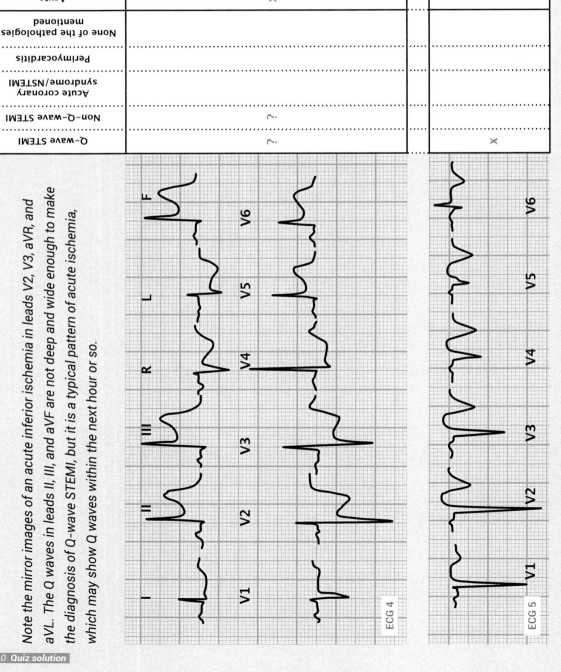

	Pathology					Phase				Which additional pathologies can be found? (use our cookbook)
	Q-wave STEMI	Non-Q-wave STEMI	Acute coronary syndrome/NSTEMI	Perimyocarditis	None of the pathologies mentioned	Acute	In resolution	Chronic (only applies to STEMI)	Nomenclature cannot be applied	
ECG 4	?	?				X				There is a helpful mirror image in V2–V4
ECG 5	X						X			

Extensive subacute anterolateral myocardial infarction (STEMI in resolution).

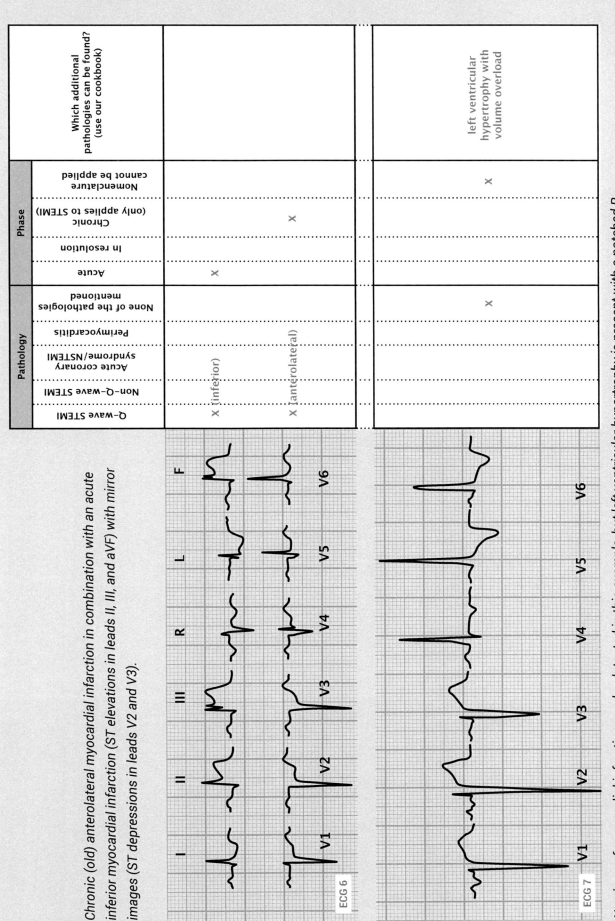

Pathology					Phase				Which additional pathologies can be found? (use our cookbook)
Q-wave STEMI	Non-Q-wave STEMI	Acute coronary syndrome/NSTEMI	Perimyocarditis	None of the pathologies mentioned	Acute	In resolution	Chronic (only applies to STEMI)	Nomenclature cannot be applied	
X (inferior)					X				
X (anterolateral)							X		
				X				X	left ventricular hypertrophy with volume overload

Chronic (old) anterolateral myocardial infarction in combination with an acute inferior myocardial infarction (ST elevations in leads II, III, and aVF) with mirror images (ST depressions in leads V2 and V3).

ECG 6

ECG 7

No signs of myocardial infarction can be detected in this example, but left ventricular hypertrophy is present with a notched R wave in lead V6 and a delayed intrinsicoid deflection (60 ms). In this case, left ventricular volume overload is probably present.

Level 10 Quiz solution

Pathology					Phase				Which additional pathologies can be found? (use our cookbook)
Q-wave STEMI	Non-Q-wave STEMI	Acute coronary syndrome NSTEMI	Perimyocarditis	None of the pathologies mentioned	Acute	In resolution	Chronic (only applies to STEMI)	Nomenclature cannot be applied	
	X				X				complete left bundle branch block
	X					X			

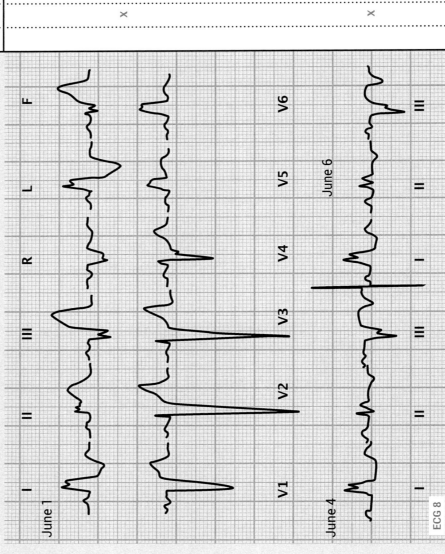

June 1 — I, II, III, R, L, F

V1, V2, V3, V4, V5, V6

June 4 — I, II, III

June 6 — I, II, III

ECG 8

This is a rare and tricky ECG: we have learned that in the case of preexisting LBBB the diagnosis of hypertrophy or myocardial infarction is impossible most of the time. However, in this example the time-dependent changes of the ST elevations in leads II, III, and aVF, and to a lesser extent in leads V5 and V6 (June 1), allow us to make the diagnosis of STEMI anyway.

We have learned that in LBBB in leads V5 and 6, we have to expect ST depression and negative T waves. Here we find a moderate ST elevation instead, which is clearly pathologic, suggesting acute coronary ischemia. Of course we may not expect any QRS signs of infarction (Q waves) because the QRS complex is already massively deformed by the BBB. This example shows you that comparison of ECGs over time can give you very important clues that you might miss otherwise!

QUIZ SOLUTION

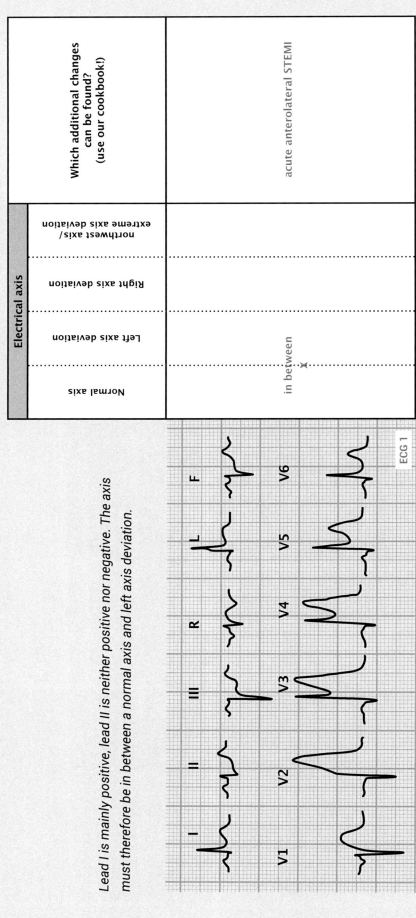

Electrical axis				Which additional changes can be found? (use our cookbook!)
Normal axis	Left axis deviation	Right axis deviation	northwest axis/ extreme axis deviation	
in between	✕			acute anterolateral STEMI

Lead I is mainly positive, lead II is neither positive nor negative. The axis must therefore be in between a normal axis and left axis deviation.

ECG 1

F
L
R
III
II
I

V6
V5
V4
V3
V2
V1

At first glance one may diagnose a right axis deviation in this example. However, something's puzzling here. The P wave and QRS complex in lead aVR are positive, which is almost never the case. Maybe this person has situs inversus? But in that case, the precordial leads would look totally different. This ECG was taken by the new medical student, so we should suspect misplacement of the extremity leads. After sending the student back to obtain another ECG, this is what he came back with:

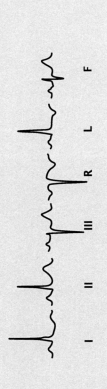

You can see that the axis is normal now. He had misplaced the electrodes (right arm and left arm) and that's what caused the right axis deviation.

Electrical axis				Which additional changes can be found? (use our cookbook!)
Normal axis	Left axis deviation	Right axis deviation	northwest axis / extreme axis deviation	
	wrong lead placement			anteroseptal STEMI in resolution

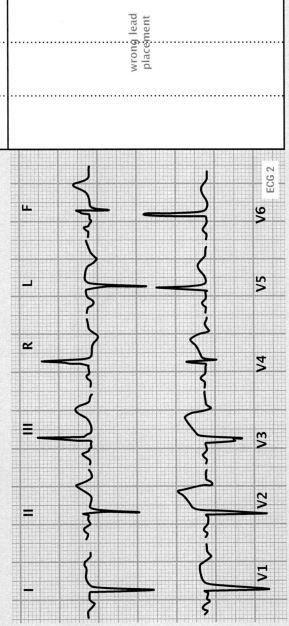

ECG 2

This example shows RBBB along with left axis deviation, indicating that the left anterior fascicle is also blocked (remember the mnemonic LAFT!). In addition, first degree AV block is also present. When bifascicular block (RBBB + block of left anterior fascicle) is combined with first degree AV block, then that's called trifascicular block, which indicates that the left posterior fascicle could also have a problem. The disturbed left ventricular repolarization may be caused by digoxin.

Electrical axis				Which additional changes can be found? (use our cookbook!)
Normal axis	Left axis deviation	Right axis deviation	northwest axis/ extreme axis deviation	
	X			RBBB plus left axis deviation = bifascicular block In addition, there is first degree AV block, so this is a case of incomplete trifascicular block

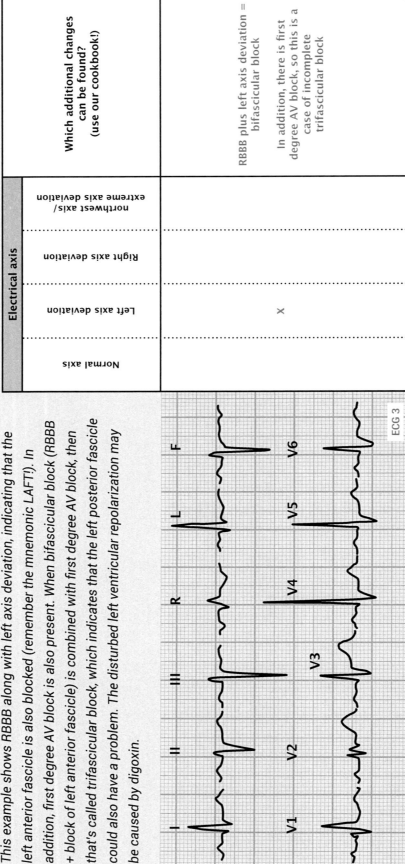

ECG 3

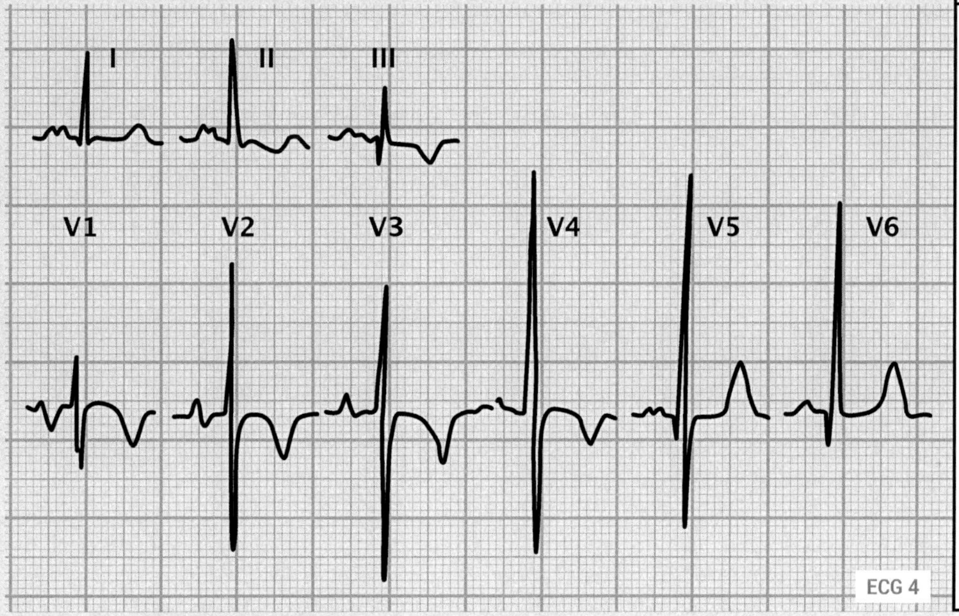

Electrical axis				Which additional changes can be found? (use our cookbook!)
Normal axis	Left axis deviation	Right axis deviation	northwest axis/ extreme axis deviation	
X				P mitrale Biventricular hypertrophy

This is a clear case of P mitrale–prolonged and biphasic in leads I, II, and III.
Also note the large negative P wave in lead V1 of more than 1 box!

ECG 4

Electrical axis				Which additional changes can be found? (use our cookbook!)
Normal axis	Left axis deviation	Right axis deviation	northwest axis/ extreme axis deviation	
X				acute inferior + lateral wall myocardial infarction + mirror image

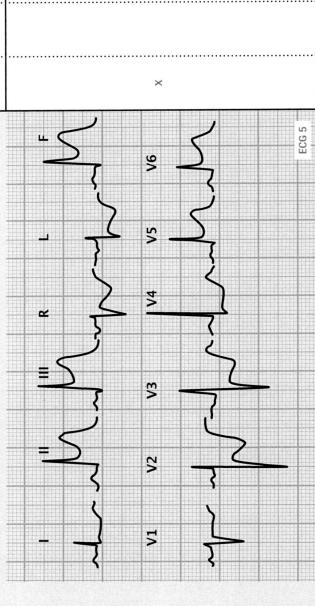

ECG 5

II III R L F

V1 V2 V3 V4 V5 V6

The tall R wave in lead V1 plus deep S wave in lead V5 point to RVH. This is supported by the high P wave in leads II and III (P pulmonale) and the right axis deviation. Even though we do not have lead aVF, we can say that with a negative QRS complex in lead I and mainly positive QRS complex in leads II and III, the axis must be right.

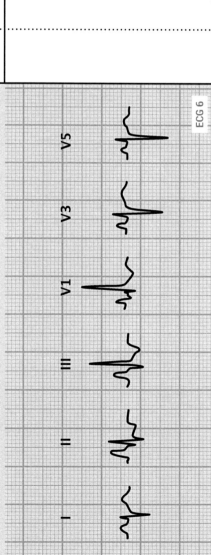

ECG 6

Electrical axis				Which additional changes can be found? (use our cookbook!)
Normal axis	Left axis deviation	Right axis deviation	northwest axis / extreme axis deviation	
		X		definite right ventricular hypertrophy
				right atrial hypertrophy

QUIZ SOLUTION

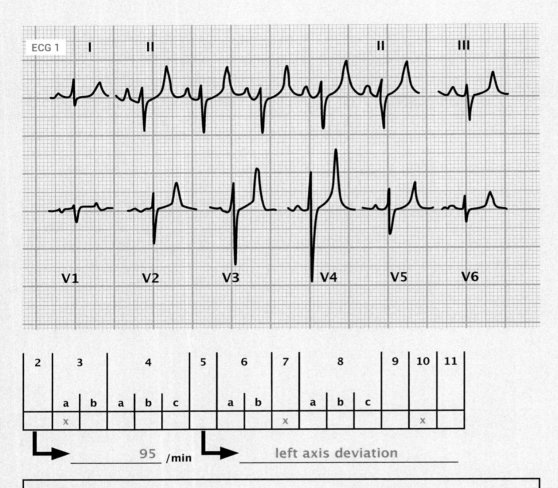

2	3		4			5	6	7	8			9	10	11
	a	b	a	b	c		a	b	a	b	c			
	x							x					x	

→ _____ 95 /min   → _____ left axis deviation _____

Diagnosis:

right atrial enlargement hypertrophy
clockwise rotation
hyperkalemia

The high P-wave amplitude in lead II of 0.3 mV is compatible with right atrial hypertrophy. The very high T waves in leads V2 to V6 could be caused by hyperkalemia. This was confirmed by a plasma potassium level of 6.5 mmol/L.

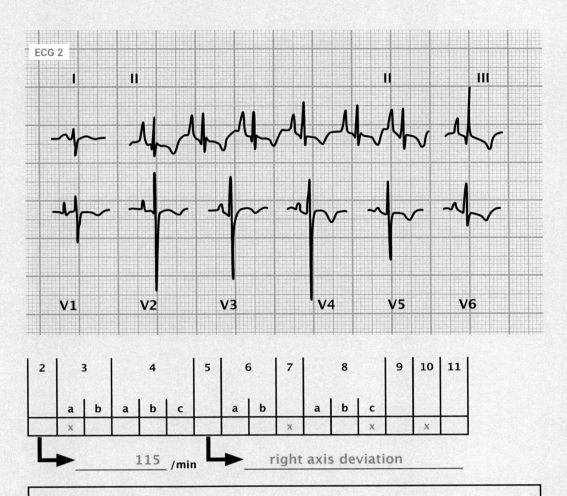

ECG 2

	I	II	II	III

V1 V2 V3 V4 V5 V6

2	3		4			5	6		7	8			9	10	11
	a	b	a	b	c		a	b		a	b	c			
	x								x			x		x	

→ _____ 115 /min → ____ right axis deviation ____

Diagnosis:

right atrial enlargement hypertrophy
clockwise rotation
right ventricular hypertrophy

Here we have clockwise rotation plus right ventricular hypertrophy. The transition zone is between leads V5 and V6, so leads V1 to V5 are over the right ventricle: clockwise rotation. The T-wave inversions from leads V1 to V6 most likely stem from right ventricular hypertrophy and are not associated with pathologic changes of the left ventricle.

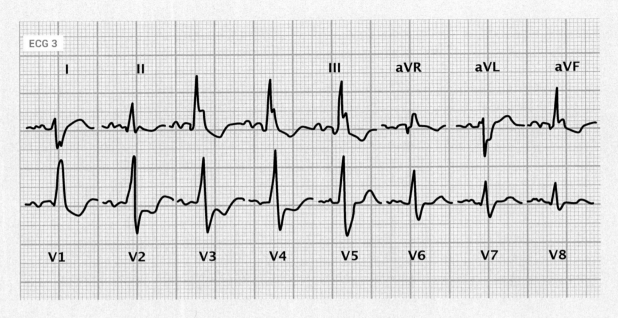

ECG 3

I II III aVR aVL aVF

V1 V2 V3 V4 V5 V6 V7 V8

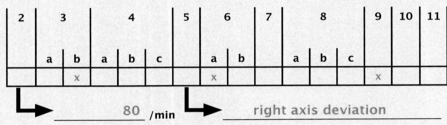

2	3		4	5	6	7	8		9	10	11
	a	b	a	b	c	a	b	a	b	c	

→ _____ 80 /min   → _____ right axis deviation _____

Diagnosis:

P mitrale
RBBB + right axis deviation = bifascicular block
chronic inferior wall myocardial infarction

The notched P wave in leads I and II is a consequence of left atrial hypertrophy (P mitrale). The right axis deviation along with the RBBB leads to the diagnosis of a left posterior fascicular block (or bifascicular block). Large Q waves (>0.04 s) in lead III and also in leads II and aVF point to the presence of old inferior wall myocardial infarction.

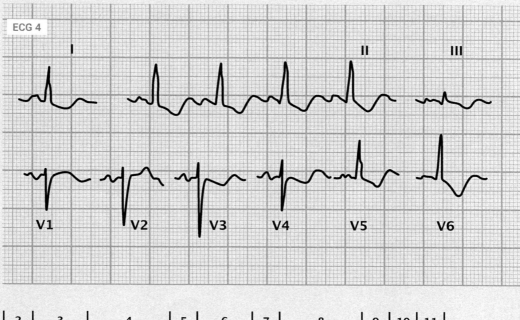

ECG 4

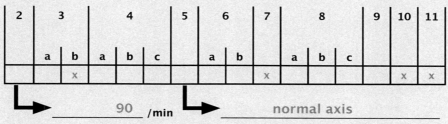

90 /min   normal axis

Diagnosis:

P mitrale
slight clockwise rotation
ST depression + U wave V3–V6
hypokalemia?

In this ECG of a patient with hypokalemia, we note the typical ST-T depression along with a prominent U wave in leads V3 and V4.

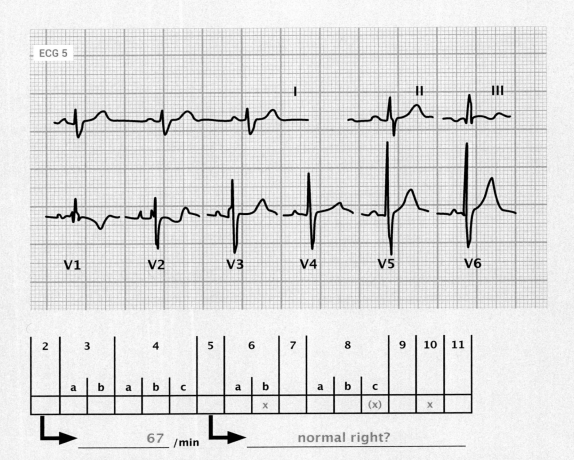

ECG 5

I   II   III

V1   V2   V3   V4   V5   V6

2	3		4			5	6	7	8			9	10	11
	a	b	a	b	c		a	b		a	b	c			
								x				(x)		x	

→ _____ 67 /min   → _____ normal right? _____

Diagnosis:

right ventricular conduction delay
(volume overload?)
possible right ventricular hypertrophy

Especially in V5 the notched QRS complex (RSRS pattern) is typical for right ventricular dilatation. Because lead I is neither clearly positive nor negative, the main vector must point exactly to +90°, i.e., just between normal and right axis.

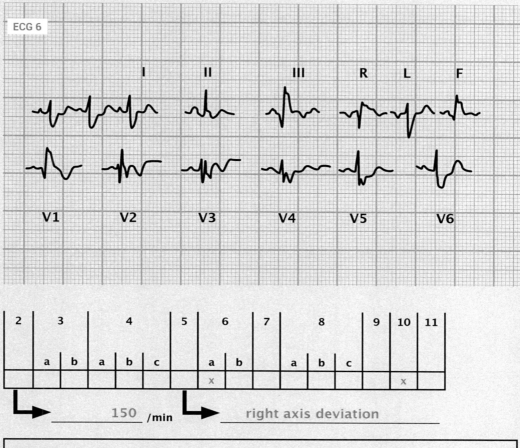

ECG 6

| | I | II | III | R | L | F |

| | V1 | V2 | V3 | V4 | V5 | V6 |

2	3		4			5	6	7	8			9	10	11
	a	b	a	b	c		a	b	a	b	c			
							x						x	

→ _____150_____ /min   → _____right axis deviation_____

Diagnosis:

PBBB

First of all, there's RBBB. In lead III, we note a pathologic Q wave and a slightly elevated ST segment, as well as T-wave inversion. This is a pattern, that would be compatible with an inferior myocardial infarction. But note that we also have a deep S wave in lead I (a so-called SIQIII pattern—typical for pulmonary embolism). Unfortunately, the patient died because of massive pulmonary embolism a few hours later.

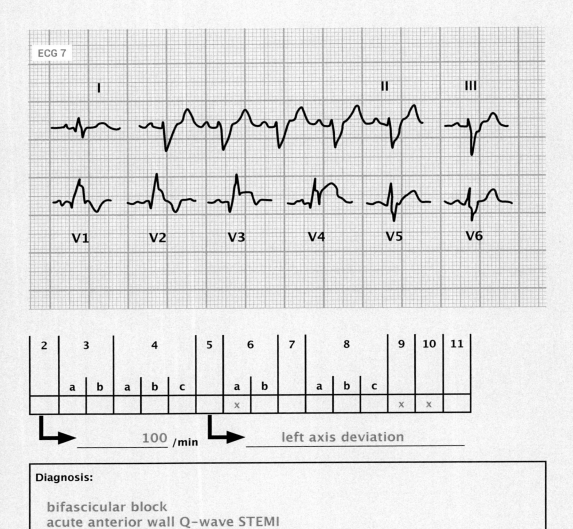

ECG 7

I   II   III

V1   V2   V3   V4   V5   V6

2	3		4			5	6		7	8			9	10	11
	a	b	a	b	c		a	b		a	b	c			
							x						x	x	

➡ _____ 100 /min   ➡   _____ left axis deviation _____

Diagnosis:

bifascicular block
acute anterior wall Q-wave STEMI

The left axis deviation along with the RBBB (bifascicular block) were caused by an anterior wall myocardial infarction leading to conduction abnormalities.

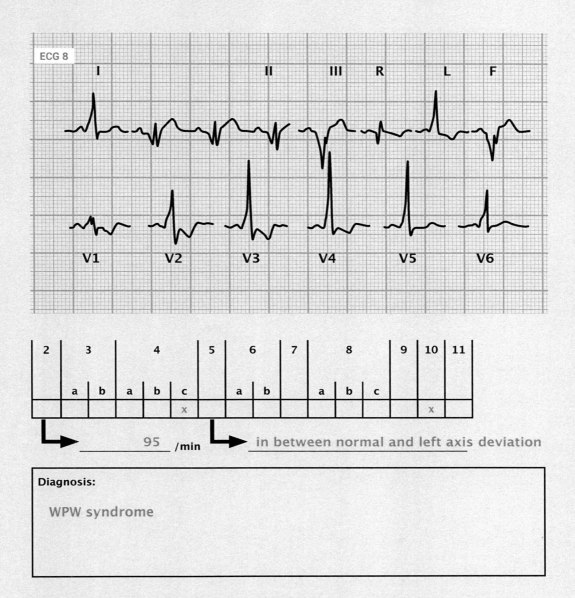

ECG 8

2	3		4			5	6		7	8			9	10	11
	a	b	a	b	c		a	b		a	b	c			
					x									x	

95 /min   in between normal and left axis deviation

Diagnosis:

WPW syndrome

The short PQ interval along with the typical delta wave in leads I, aVL, and V2 to V6 lead to the diagnosis of WPW syndrome. Remember that after the diagnosis of WPW syndrome has been established, no additional disturbances of repolarization or pathologic Q waves must be diagnosed.

Level 13

QUIZ SOLUTION

Sinus		Heart rate	If there is sinus rhythm, make additional diagnoses according to our cookbook.
no	yes		
X		~105	flattening of T waves in lead I

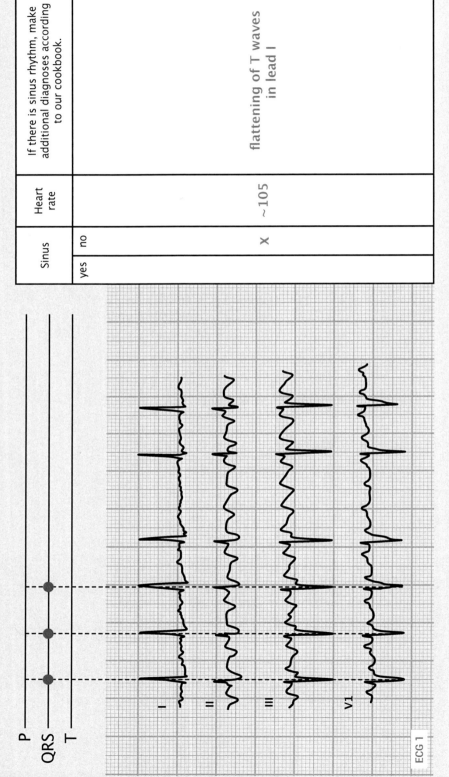

P
QRS
T

ECG 1

I
II
III
v1

We can find P waves in this example. However, there's not only one P wave in front of each QRS complex but several of them. Furthermore, we can't really tell whether P waves are positive or negative in lead II. So there are a couple of reasons why this can't be sinus rhythm.

Sinus		Heart rate	If there is sinus rhythm, make additional diagnoses according to our cookbook.
no			
yes	X	75	P mitrale (most pro-minently seen in V1). First degree AV block (PR 0.24 s) with left axis deviation and RBBB (i.e., trifascicular block).

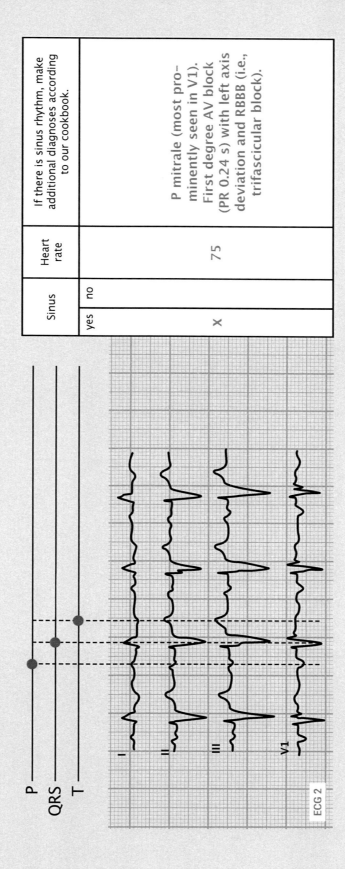

P

QRS

T

I

II

III

V1

ECG 2

Sinus		Heart rate	If there is sinus rhythm, make additional diagnoses according to our cookbook.
no			
yes		~75	flattening of T waves in lead I
	x		

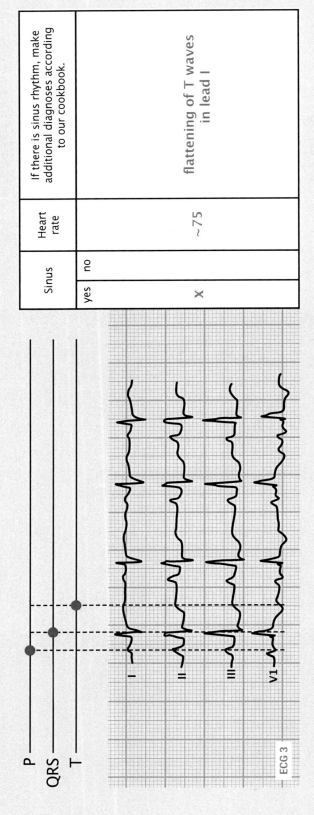

P

QRS

T

I

II

III

V1

ECG 3

Sinus rhythm doesn't always have to be completely rhythmic as we can see in this example. The RR intervals are different from beat to beat in this case (maximum RR interval: 0.84 s, minimum RR interval: 0.68 s). This is called sinus arrhythmia. Furthermore, there are signs of right atrial enlargement (P pulmonale), and the axis is right in between a normal axis and right axis deviation. The notching in lead V1 (without RBBB) is indicative of right ventricular volume overload.

Sinus		Heart rate	If there is sinus rhythm, make additional diagnoses according to our cookbook.
no	yes		
X		~500 ?	

P ——————————
QRS ——————————
T ——————————

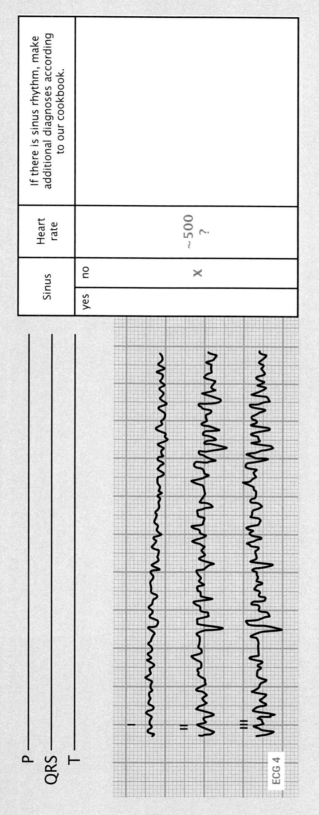

ECG 4

Completely irregular tracing. No distinct curves can be identified. This can't be sinus rhythm.

Sinus		Heart rate	If there is sinus rhythm, make additional diagnoses according to our cookbook.
yes	no		
x		~145	

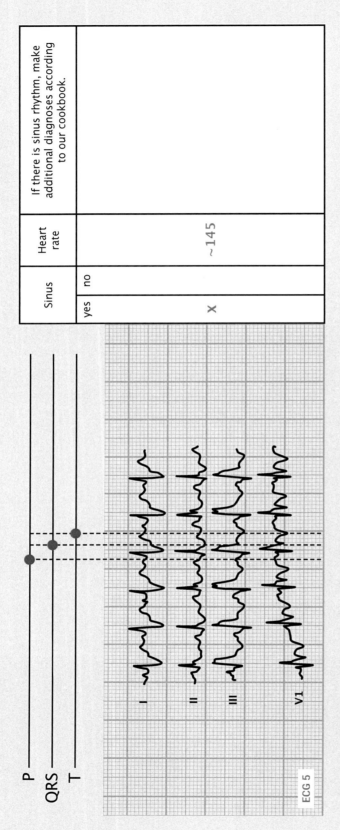

P

QRS

T

I

II

III

v1

ECG 5

This is sinus rhythm with a heart rate of 145 beats/min, which is also called sinus tachycardia. The axis is right between a normal axis and right axis deviation. The QRS complex is widened to 0.14 s, and with the RSRS pattern in lead V1 we can diagnose RBBB. This was a young man presenting to the ER in shock with massive pulmonary embolism. He died shortly thereafter. Notice the typical SIQIII pattern as in a previous example!

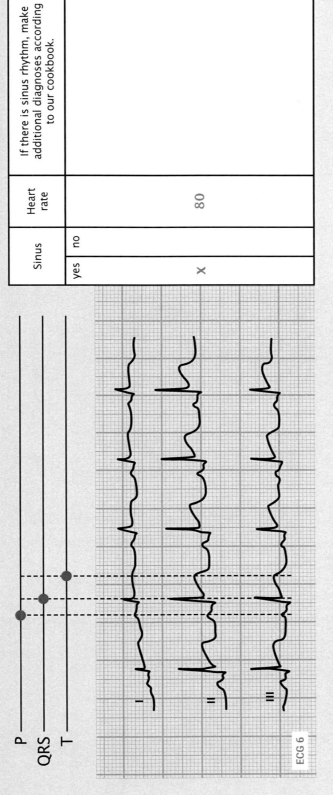

Sinus		Heart rate	If there is sinus rhythm, make additional diagnoses according to our cookbook.
no			
yes	X	80	

ECG 6

Normal axis. ST elevation in leads II and III but also in lead I. There are no Q waves. This could be (1) perimyocarditis, or (2) acute ischemia. In fact, this patient had STEMI, the extent of which was much better seen in the precordial leads, and he was treated by stent placement.

Sinus		Heart rate	If there is sinus rhythm, make additional diagnoses according to our cookbook.
yes	no		
	x	280	

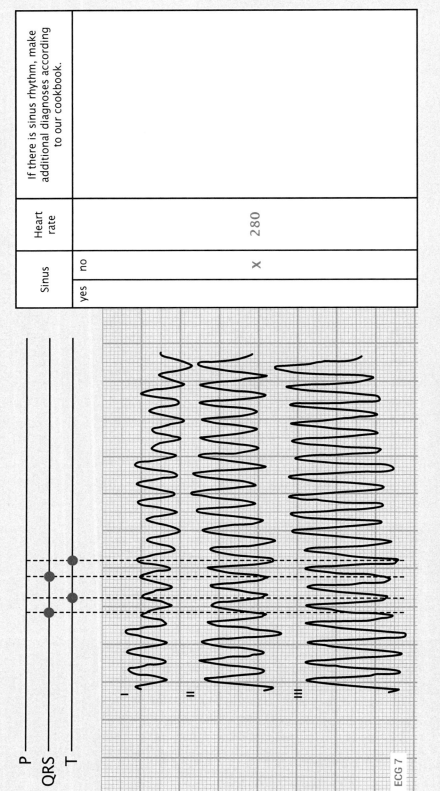

P

QRS

T

ECG 7

No P waves are visible in this tracing. This cannot be sinus rhythm.

Sinus		Heart rate	If there is sinus rhythm, make additional diagnoses according to our cookbook.
no			
yes	x	47	

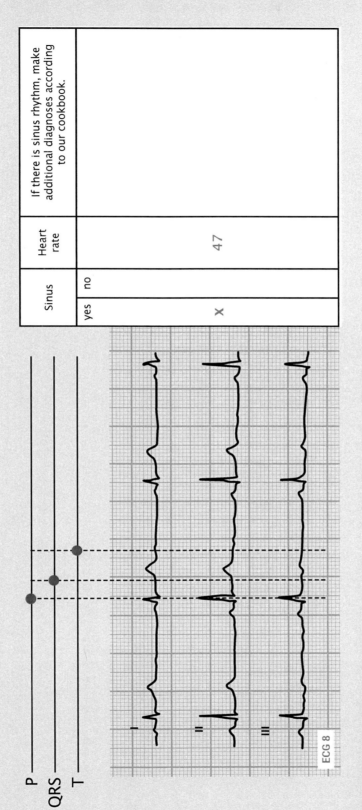

P ———

QRS ———

T ———

ECG 8

Sinus rhythm with a heart rate of <50 beats/min is called sinus bradycardia. The axis is normal. Sinus bradycardia does not have to be pathologic. To the contrary, it can be a sign of good physical fitness. In older individuals, sinus bradycardia (without adequate response to exertion) can cause problems like dizziness and falls and can even lead to pacemaker implantation.

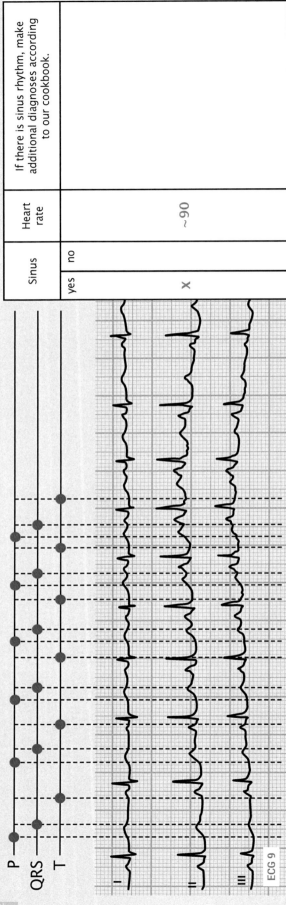

Sinus		Heart rate	If there is sinus rhythm, make additional diagnoses according to our cookbook.
no	yes		
	X	~90	

ECG 9

P
QRS
T

I
II
III

The heart rate in this patient with sinus rhythm varies between 70 and 100 beats/min. There seems to be a pattern...heart rate is slower in the beginning of the tracing, gets faster, and slows down again at the end. This type of sinus arrhythmia is called respiratory sinus arrhythmia (heart rate increases on inspiration and decreases on expiration). This form of ar-rhythmia is very common in young individuals and is not pathologic. Also, the axis changes slightly with respiration.

Sinus		Heart rate	If there is sinus rhythm, make additional diagnoses according to our cookbook.
no	yes		
x		70	

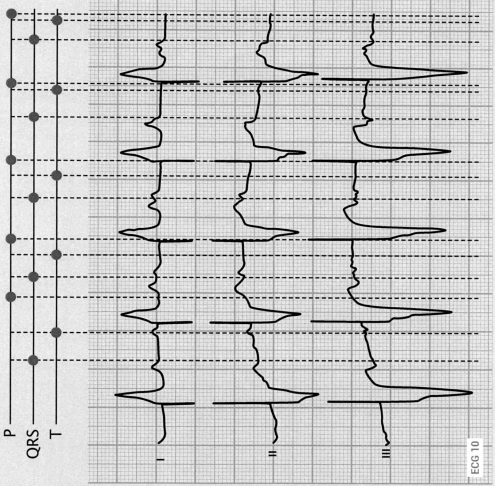

ECG 10

There are P waves in this tracing, but they do not occur at a fixed interval before each QRS complex. So this cannot be sinus rhythm.

P
QRS
T

I
II
III

INDEX

A

Abnormal ECG, patterns in
  M pattern, 41
  notching, 41
  in V1 or V2, 40
  in V5 or V6, 40
ACS. *See* Acute coronary syndromes
Acute anterior wall Q-wave STEMI, 204
Acute coronary syndromes, 186, 187
  causes of, 92
  non-STEMI, 92
    characterization of, 93
    in LAD, 95
    symptoms, 94
  stages of, 93
  with ST elevation, 94
  STEMI, 92
    characterization of, 93
  unstable angina, 92
    characterization of, 93
    symptoms, 93
  without ST elevation, 94–95
Acute inferior ischemia, 188
Acute ischemic event, 187
Acute myocardial infarction, 186
Amplitude measurement, 14
  and isoelectric line, 15
  quiz on, 17–18
  S-wave, 16
Anterior wall myocardial infarction, 204
Anterolateral changes, 32
Anteroseptal changes, 32
Anteroseptal infarct, 176
Atrial depolarization, 8
  and P-wave duration, 22
Atrial enlargement and P-wave duration, 22
Atrial hypertrophy
  evaluation of, 116
  left, 116
  right, 116
Atrial repolarization, 8

Augmented leads, 83
AV block I. *See* First degree atrioventricular block
aVF lead, 83
  and vectors, 109
    mainly negative, 111
    mainly positive, 110
aVL lead, 83
aVR lead, 83

B

Bifascicular block, 114, 194, 200, 204
Biventricular hypertrophy, 195

C

Cabrera system, 107
Calibration, 14
Cardiac axis
  abnormalities of, 106–107
  case studies for assessing
    left ventricular hypertrophy and right axis deviation, 115
    right ventricular hypertrophy and right axis deviation, 115
    ventricular depolarization, 113–114
  definition of, 106
  left axis deviation. *See* Left axis deviation
  normal axis. *See* Normal axis
  quiz on, 120–125
  right axis deviation. *See* Right axis deviation
  way to determine, 106
    aVF and vectors. *See* aVF
    lead I and vectors. *See* Lead I and vectors
    lead II and vectors. *See* Lead II and vectors
Cellular potassium loss, 128–129
Chest pain, 95
Clockwise rotation, 198, 199
Complete bundle branch block, 24, 25–26, 41, 44–45, 157–159, 181
Complete left bundle branch block, 44–47, 161–165, 190
Complete right bundle branch block, 44–47, 161–165
Counterclockwise rotation, 166–171, 181

D

Definite right ventricular hypertrophy, 197
Delta wave, 24, 161–165, 175
    quiz on, 44–47
Depolarization of ventricles, 8, 50
    complete bundle branch block and, 41
    and PR interval, 23
    and QRS duration, 24
Drowning in negativity, 70

E

ECG evaluation
    isoelectric line. *See* Isoelectric line
    quiz on, 87–89
    right ventricular hypertrophy assessment, 52
    step-by-step approach for, 85–86
    ST segment, 96, 98
ECG grid
    amplitude measurement, 14
    time measurement, 15–16
ECG machines, print speed of, 15
ECG wave, 50
Electrical axis, 192–197
Electrical vector, 50
Extreme axis deviation, 192–197

F

First degree atrioventricular block, 23, 207
    PR interval, 118, 131, 141
    quiz on, 25–26, 157–159

H

Heart rate, 141, 212–213
    evaluation, 130–131, 133–137
    and QT time, 129
Hypercalcemia, QT interval in, 129
Hyperkalemia, 198
    ECG changes associated with, 128
Hypocalcemia, QT interval in, 129
Hypokalemia, 201
    ECG changes associated with, 128–129

I

Incomplete bundle branch block, 41
Inferior myocardial infarction, 203
Inferior wall myocardial infarction
    changes in, 83
    direct electrical image of, 84
Intercostal space, finding and counting, 31
Interval measurement. *See* Time measurement
Isoelectric line
    and amplitude measurement, 15
    definition of, 8, 60
    P-wave, 15
    QRS complex, 15
    QT interval, 16
    S-wave, 16
    and time measurement, 15

L

LAF. *See* Left anterior fascicle
Lateral wall, changes of, 83
LBB. *See* Left bundle branch
LBBB. *See* Left bundle branch block
Lead I and vectors
    mainly negative, 109, 110, 111
    mainly positive, 108, 109
    negative deflection, 107
    positive deflection, 107
Lead II and vectors
    mainly negative, 109
    mainly positive, 108
Leads
    information provided by, 160
    precordial. *See* Precordial leads
    ventricle represented by, 160
Left anterior fascicle, 113, 194
    bifascicular block involving, 114
Left atrial hypertrophy, 116
    and P mitrale, 117
Left axis deviation, 112, 192–197
    and LAF(T) block, 114
    and RBBB, 207
Left bundle branch, 113
Left bundle branch block, 172, 191

M pattern of, 41
negative T waves in, 62
QRS complex broadening in, 114
QRS duration in, 41, 43
ST depressions in, 62
Left posterior fascicle, 113
Left ventricular hypertrophy, 166–171, 174, 176, 182
assessment using Sokolow index, 51–52
QRS amplitude, 118, 131, 141
quiz on, 53–57
and right axis deviation, 115
R/S ratios, 53–57
R waves, 53–57
S waves, 53–57
with volume overload, 189
Left ventricular volume overload, 166–171
R/S ratios, 53–57
R waves, 53–57
S waves, 53–57
LGL syndrome. *See* Lown-Ganong-Levine syndrome
Limb leads, 30
components of, 83
frontal plane, 82
recording, 83
wires, 83
Lown-Ganong-Levine syndrome, 24
PR interval, 118, 131, 141
quiz on, 25–26, 157–159
Low voltage, 117
QRS amplitude, 118, 131, 141
LPF. *See* Left posterior fascicle

M

Main vector, 106
Mirror images, 84
Momentary vectors, 106
Myocardial aneurysm, 94
Myocardial infarction, 181, 183–185, 196
at anterolateral region, 73
chronic inferior wall, 200
chronic phase and T wave, 94

effect on QRS complex, 76–79, 92, 177–180, 186
drowning in negativity, 70
Q wave, 70, 72–74
R wave, 71, 74–75
QRS infarction signs, 118, 131
subacute phase and ST segment, 94
Myocardial ischemia, 176
Myocardial scarring, 85

N

Non–Q-wave infarction, 94
and Q-wave, 85
Non–Q-wave STEMI, 188, 190
Normal axis, 108, 112, 192–197, 210
Normal ECG, 40
Northwest axis, 111, 112, 113
Northwest axis deviation, 192–197
NSTEMI, 187

P

Paper speed and time measurement, 15
Pathologic Q waves, 177–180, 181, 203
criteria for, 72, 84
infarct at anterolateral region, 73
infarct in V4 and V5 area, 72–73
Perimyocarditis, 186, 210
and ST elevation, 95–96
P mitrale, 25–26, 116, 157–159, 195, 200, 207
Posterolateral changes, 32
P pulmonale, 116
Precordial leads
anatomical regions depicted by
basal septum, 31
LV anterior wall, 32
LV lateral wall, 32
LV posterior wall, 32
right ventricle, 31
appearance of, 73
ECG pattern
quiz on, 37
R/S ratio, 33–35
transitional zone, 35–36

and electrical axis, 192–197
functions of, 30
horizontal plane, 82
location on Cabrera circle and vector
   lead I, 107–108
   lead II, 108
normal appearance of, 40
placement of, 30
and QRS duration. *See* QRS duration
starting with initial R wave, 74
Preexcitation syndrome, 23
Premature ventricular beats, 62
PR interval, 97, 141, 154–156, 183–185
   evaluation of, 86, 154
   first AV block, 118, 131, 141
   LGL syndrome, 118, 131, 141
   WPW syndrome, 118, 131, 141
PR interval duration, 161–165
   AV block I and, 23
   normal values, 23
   and preexcitation syndrome, 23–24
   quiz on, 44–47
Prinzmetal angina, 95
Pulmonary embolism, 203
P waves, 8, 141, 152, 153, 206
   amplitude measurement, 17–18
   duration of, 22, 154–156
   identifying, 9–10
   interval measurement, 15, 17–18
   and left atrial hypertrophy, 116–118, 131, 141
   and right atrial hypertrophy, 116–118, 131, 141

Q

QRS amplitude, 97
   evaluation of, 86
   left ventricular hypertrophy, 118, 131, 141
   low voltage, 118, 131, 141
   right ventricular hypertrophy, 118, 131, 141
QRS axis, 118, 131
QRS complexes, 152, 175, 181
   abnormal patterns in
      M pattern, 41
      notching, 41

      V1 or V2, 40
      V5 or V6, 40
   amplitude measurement, 17–18
   broadening, 114
   definition of, 8
   distance between, 130
   drowning in negativity, 70
   duration of, 161–165
   identifying components of, 9–10
   interval measurement, 15, 17–18
      lengthening of interval, 24
   lengthening of, 24
   LGL syndrome and, 24
   sharpest waves, 152–153
   WPW syndrome and, 24
QRS duration, 97, 154–156, 183–185
   complete/incomplete BBB, 118, 131
   in complete LBBB, 41
   in complete RBBB, 42
   evaluation of, 86, 154–155
   and incomplete bundle branch block, 41
   lengthened in WPW syndrome, 42–43
   quiz on, 44–47
QRS infarction signs, 97
   evaluation of, 86
   myocardial infarction, 118, 131
QRS shape, 161–165
QS pattern, 177–180
QTc time, 129
QT duration, 132, 154
QT interval, 154–156
   approaches to assess, 130
   corrected. *See* QTc time
   and heart rate, 129
   in hypercalcemia, 129
   in hypocalcemia, 129
   in hypokalemia, 129
   interval measurement, 16–18
Q waves, 74, 188
   and non–Q-wave infarctions, 85
   progression in leads V4 to V6, 72
Q-wave STEMI, 188–189

R

RBB. *See* Right bundle branch

RBBB. *See* Right bundle branch block

Repolarization, 8, 174

Respiratory sinus arrhythmia, 213

Revascularization and ST elevation, 94

Right atrial enlargement, 208

Right atrial hypertrophy, 116, 197, 198, 199

  and P pulmonale, 117

  and P wave, 116

Right axis deviation, 110, 112, 113, 192–197

  and left ventricular hypertrophy, 115

  and right bundle branch block, 114

  and right ventricular hypertrophy, 115

Right bundle branch, 113

Right bundle branch block, 181, 203, 204

  with block of LPF, 114

  with left anterior hemiblock, 114

  and left axis deviation, 194, 207

  left fascicle blocked in, 114

  M pattern of, 42

  negative T waves in, 62

  QRS complex broadening in, 114

  QRS duration of, 42

  and right axis deviation, 114, 200

  ST depressions in, 62

Right ventricular conduction delay, 163, 202

Right ventricular hypertrophy, 166–171, 174, 199, 202

  assessment of, 52

  QRS amplitude, 118

  quiz on, 53–57

  and right axis deviation, 115

  R/S ratios, 53–57

  R waves, 53–57

  S waves, 53–57

Right ventricular volume overload, 166–171, 208

  R/S ratios, 53–57

  R waves, 53–57

  S waves, 53–57

Rotation, 86, 97, 118, 131, 141, 166–171, 183–185

RR intervals, 130, 208

RRS right ventricular hypertrophy, 52

R/S ratios

  left ventricular hypertrophy, 53–57

  left ventricular volume overload, 53–57

  right ventricular hypertrophy, 53–57

  right ventricular volume overload, 53–57

RSRS pattern, 210

RSS criteria, 52

R wave, 50–51, 74, 177–180

  amplitude and myocardial infarction, 74–75

  changes in morphology of, 41

  left ventricular hypertrophy, 53–57

  left ventricular volume overload, 53–57

  right ventricular hypertrophy, 53–57

  right ventricular volume overload, 53–57

  size of, 50

  in V5 or V6, 51

S

Sinus arrhythmia, 208

Sinus bradycardia, 212

Sinus rhythm, 208, 209–210, 211–212

  criteria for, 140–141

  determining, 143–149

Sinus tachycardia, 210

Sokolow index, 51–52, 171, 173

Standard leads, 83

ST depression, 60, 172–176, 175

  forms of, 61, 63–66, 119

  in hypokalemia, 129

  and U wave, 201

ST elevation, 119, 175

  ACS with, 94

  ACS without, 94–95

  perimyocarditis and, 95–96

  with Q waves, 94

  and revascularization, 94

  vagotonia and, 96

  variant angina and, 95

Sternal angle, 31

ST segment, 60, 92, 186–187

  elevation of, 93

  evaluation of, 96, 98–103

resolution, 94
ST-T depression, 201
ST-T segment, 98, 119, 132, 141
S waves, 50–51
  interval measurement, 16
  left ventricular hypertrophy, 53–57
  left ventricular volume overload, 53–57
  right ventricular hypertrophy, 53–57
  right ventricular volume overload, 53–57
  in V1 or V2, 51

T

Time measurement, 15–16
  and isoelectric line, 15
  and paper speed, 15
  P-wave, 15
  QRS complex, 15
  QT interval, 16
  quiz on, 17–18
  S-wave, 16
T negativity. See T-wave inversions
Transition zone of heart and rotation, 118, 131, 141
Trifascicular block, 207
Troponin, 93
T–U waves, 132
T-wave inversions, 60, 172–176, 183, 187, 199, 203
  asymmetric, 62
  biphasic, 62
  patterns of, 62–66
  specificity for coronary artery disease, 62
  symmetric, 62
T waves, 8, 60, 152, 153, 175
  biphasic, 154, 172
  flattening of, 206, 208
  in hyperkalemia, 128
  in hypokalemia, 129
  identifying, 9–10
  terminally negative biphasic, 176
  in vagotonia, 128

U

U wave in hypokalemia, 129

V

Vagotonia
  and ST elevation, 96
  T wave in, 128
Variant angina. See Prinzmetal angina
Vectorcardiography, 106
Ventricular depolarization, 106
Voltage measurement. See Amplitude measurement
Volume overload, 41, 202
  left ventricle, 161–165
  left ventricular, 44–47, 53–57
  right ventricle, 161–165
  right ventricular, 44–47, 53–57

W

Wolff-Parkinson-White syndrome, 24, 62, 161–165, 175, 184, 205
  PR interval, 118, 131, 141
  QRS duration lengthened in, 42–43
  quiz on, 25–26, 44–47, 157–159
WPW syndrome. See Wolff-Parkinson-White syndrome

22868791R00128